Multiple Choice Questions in

PATHOLOGY

With answers and explanations

Third Edition

I. L. Brown
Lecturer in Pathology, University of Glasgow;
Honorary Consultant Pathologist, Greater Glasgow Health Board,
Glasgow, Scotland

Edward Arnold
A division of Hodder & Stoughton
LONDON MELBOURNE AUCKLAND

230459

© 1992 Edward Arnold

First published in Great Britain 1992

British Library Cataloguing in Publication Data

Brown I.L.
   Multiple Choice Questions in Pathology:
   With Answers and Explanatory Comments
   3 Rev. ed
   I. Title
   616.07076

ISBN 0-340-55164-x

Whilst the advice and information in this book is believed to be true and accurate at the date of going to press, neither the author nor the publisher can accept any legal responsibility or liability for any errors or omissions that may be made. In particular (but without limiting the generality of the preceding disclaimer) every effort has been made to check drug dosages; however, it is still possible that errors have been missed. Furthermore, dosage schedules are constantly being revised and new side-effects recognized. For these reasons the reader is strongly urged to consult the drug companies' printed instructions before administering any of the drugs recommended in this book.

Typeset in Univers Light by Anneset. Printed and bound in Great Britain for Edward Arnold, a division of Hodder and Stoughton Limited, Mill Road, Dunton Green, Sevenoaks, Kent TN13 2YA by R Clay (St. Ives plc), Bungay, Suffolk.

- (IAN 1993

Contents

Introduction

The use of multiple choice questions (MCQs) for examinations in pathology is almost universal in our Medical Schools. A number of books are available giving students the opportunity to practise MCQ examination technique, and to test their knowledge as an aid to revision. Those books that contain explanations of the answers are more useful as learning aids.

This 3rd edition of Multiple Choice Questions in Pathology is derived from the new 13th Edition of Muirs Textbook of Pathology, which has been completely revised and rewritten. In the light of the revision of Muir the opportunity has been taken to rewrite the questions relating to general pathology to include the recent advances in molecular pathology and cell biology, which are now part of the undergraduate curriculum in Pathology.

As in the previous editions the questions are arranged in sections directly related to the chapters in Muir enabling the student to follow up the explanatory comments by going direct to the relevant chapter in Muir. Although the book may be used along with Muir this is not necessary since the explanatory comments are detailed enough for revision purposes.

A further difference from previous editions is the inclusion of **True/False** questions in the general pathology section. Many examinations include this type of question and so will allow students to practise the different technique required for these.

How to use the book. There are four different types of question:
  (i) A direct question is asked in the stem and a choice is made from five alternatives.
  (ii) A list of five alternatives is given from which the most appropriate association for each of a list of three conditions should be chosen.
  (iii) A list of five steps in a pathological process is given and the fourth step in chronological order is to be indicated.
  (iv) A set of five statements regarding a topic is given and each has to be described as true or false.

The answers and explanations are given directly opposite the questions on the facing page. It is advisable to complete the whole page or a whole section before revealing the answers.

Marking systems for MCQs vary from Medical School to Medical School – apply your own system for an assessment of your knowledge, but remember that in **True/False** questions the counter-mark is always a full mark off, so guessing is not recommended!

1   For each of the features on the left select the most appropriate association from
     the list on the right.
     a. Dedifferentiation   A. Development of a clone of cells
     b. Heterotopia   growing independently of normal
     c. Metaplasia   cellular controls
                                            B. Loss of cell specialisation
                                            C. Result of error in
                                                intercellular communication in
                                                the fetus
                                            D. Result of gene activation due
                                                to environmental change
                                            E. Structural and functional
                                                specialisation of cells

2   For each example of necrosis listed on the left select the most suitable
     description from those on the right.
     a. Caseous necrosis   A. Cheese-like material
     b. Coagulative necrosis   B. Dull, swollen firm area
     c. Colliquative necrosis   C. Firm yellow/white patches
                                            D. Green/black discolouration
                                            E. Soft, liquefying material

3   For each of the features of DNA replication listed on the left select the most
     appropriate association from the list on the right.
     a. Splicing   A. Modulation of promoter activity
     b. Transcription   B. mRNA copy of DNA
     c. Translation   C. Production of polypeptide chains
                                                from tRNA
                                            D. Removal of superfluous introns
                                            E. Stretches of DNA nearer 3' end
                                                of chain

4   For each of the patterns of inheritance on the left select the most appropriate
     disease from those on the right.
     a. Autosomal dominant   A. Ankylosing spondylitis
     b. Autosomal recessive   B. Breast cancer
     c. X-linked recessive   C. Duchenne muscular dystrophy
                                            D. Mucopolysaccharidosis
                                            E. Neurofibromatosis

1 **a = B** Loss of specialisation may be seen as changes in cytology or function of cells and tissues.

  b = C Groups of cells differentiate in a way which is inappropriate to their anatomical localisation.

  c = D This is the change of one differentiated cell type into another, and is often seen as a result of environmental factors, e.g. cigarette smoking.

    Structural and functional specialisation of cells is differentiation (E), and A is a possible definition of neoplasia.

2 **a = A** This is the typical appearance of tuberculous necrosis, but a similar appearance may also be seen in necrotic tumours, particularly squamous carcinoma.

  b = B This is typical of infarction in solid organs, such as heart and kidney. Histologically 'ghost' outlines of the tissue structure are still visible.

  c = E This is typical of necrotic tissue with a high content of fluid, e.g. brain. Histologically the tissue architecture is lost.

3 **a = D** Superfluous information transcribed from the introns of the genes is edited out of the mRNA in this process.

  b = B Transcription is the process whereby an mRNA copy of the DNA of the gene is produced before a polypeptide can be synthesised.

  c = C mRNA produces tRNA, with the tRNA amino acids arranged in the order necessary for the production of the specified polypeptide.

    Promoters (E) control transcription by acting as switches upstream to the gene to be transcribed.

    Modulation of promoter activity (A) is undertaken by an enhancer, which is a separate regulatory element on the same DNA molecule.

4 **a = D** A specific enzyme deficiency results in excessive accumulation of mucopolysaccharide in the viscera.

  b = E A dominant character is expressed in one parent and can be expected in half of the offspring; multiple tumours of small nerves are present in this condition.

  c = C The gene for this form of muscular dystrophy is present on the X-chromosome, hence females are not affected (having one normal X-chromosome).

    Ankylosing spondylitis is a disease of the vertebral column, which is associated with specific HLA type (A).

    Breast cancer (B) may occur with increased frequency in particular families but without a genetic component.

5   For each of the features of the clotting (coagulation) mechanism on the left
     select the most appropriate association from the list on the right.
     a. Common pathway   A. Can occur in the test-tube
     b. Extrinsic pathway   B. Converts prothrombin to thrombin
     c. Intrinsic pathway   C. Produced by fibroblasts
                                      D. Production of plasmin
                                      E. Result of tissue injury

6   Which *one* of the following is *not* associated with thrombosis?
     A. Activation of the coagulation mechanism
     B. Endothelial damage
     C. Formation of platelet aggregates
     D. Thrombocytopenia
     E. Vascular stasis

7   Which *one* of the following is *not* a feature of thromboxane A_2?
     A. Inhibits platelet adenyl cyclase
     B. Produced by action of an endothelial cell enzyme
     C. Produced by conversion of cyclic endoperoxidase by
        platelets
     D. Prostaglandin with a half-life of 30 seconds
     E. Stimulates platelet adhesion and aggregation

8   If the following events were placed in chronological order which would come
     fourth?
     A. Cholecystectomy
     B. Deep venous thrombosis
     C. Embolization
     D. Pulmonary infarction
     E. Stasis in calf veins

9   For each of the types of infarct listed on the left select the most suitable cause
     from the list on the right.
     a. Cerebral boundary   A. Coronary artery thrombosis
        zone infarction   B. Embolization of renal artery
     b. Haemorrhagic infarction   C. Follows an episode of
     c. Venous infarction   hypotension
                                      D. Marantic thrombosis of superior
                                         longitudinal sinus
                                      E. Obstruction of superior
                                         mesenteric artery

5   **a = B**   The common pathway (produced by extrinsic or intrinsic routes) results in the conversion of prothrombin (factor II) to thrombin (factor IIa), which converts fibrinogen (factor I) to fibrin monomer.

    b = E   The extrinsic pathway is the result of the action of thrombokinase produced by tissue injury.

    c = A   The intrinsic pathway results in clotting without the participation of tissue injury factors.
    The production of plasmin (D) is the result of activators on plasminogen and is responsible for the solubilisation of fibrin. Fibrin is not produced by fibroblasts (C).

6   **D**   Lack of platelets or abnormal platelets will result in a decreased ability to form thrombus.
    The major factors predisposing to thrombosis are abnormalities of vessel walls (B), disturbances of blood flow (E) and alterations to blood, which favour coagulation (A) and platelet aggregation (C).

7   **B**   Vascular endothelium is rich in prostacyclin synthetase, which produces prostacyclin from the cyclic endoperoxides. Thromboxane A_2 is produced by the action of platelet thromboxane synthetase on cyclic endoperoxides (C). It stimulates platelet adhesion and aggregation (E) by inhibiting platelet adenyl cyclase (A). It is a prostaglandin with a very short half-life (D).

8   **C**   During surgery and postoperatively (A) stasis occurs in the deep veins of the calves (E) resulting in thrombosis (B); fragments of thrombus break off into the circulation (C), plug the pulmonary arteries and cause infarction (D). A significant number of emboli come from thrombosis of the pelvic veins.

9   **a = C**   There are areas of relatively poor vascularisation between the territories of the major cerebral arteries; hypotension may result in poor perfusion in these areas giving localised infarction.

    b = E   Obstruction of the superior mesenteric artery results in haemorrhagic infarction of the intestine, which progresses to gangrene.

    c = D   In debilitated children thrombosis of the superior longitudinal sinus results in engorgement of the cerebral cortical veins.
    Emboli in the renal artery cause pale wedge-shaped infarcts of the renal cortex (B). Thrombosis of the coronary arteries results in myocardial infarction (A).
    Both of these are examples of end arteries.

10 For each of the types of shock listed on the left select the most appropriate
    cause from the list on the right.
    a. Cardiogenic shock   A. Burns involving 15% of the skin
    b. Hypovolaemic shock   surface
    c. Septic shock   B. Cytotoxic drug therapy
                                        C. Incompatible blood transfusion
                                        D. Pancreatitis
                                        E. Rupture of heart valve cusp

11 If the following features of the acute inflammatory reaction were placed in
    chronological order which would come *fourth*?
    A. Arteriolar contraction
    B. Blood flow slows
    C. Dilatation of arterioles
    D. Emigration of leucocytes from blood vessels
    E. Protein-rich fluid escapes from blood vessels

12 Which *one* of the following ultrastructural features is believed to allow for the
    increased permeability of the vascular endothelium in acutely inflamed tissue?
    A. Cytoplasmic pinocytotic vesicles
    B. Gaps in endothelial tight junctions
    C. Gaps in basement membrane
    D. Increase in number of phagolysosomes
    E. No morphological changes

13 For each of the phases of increased vascular permeability in the acute
    inflammatory reaction noted on the left choose the most suitable association
    from those on the right
    a. Immediate sustained   A. Endothelial cells elongate
       response   B. Primarily a response to histamine
    b. Immediate transient   C. Response to a mild degree of
       response   physical injury
    c. Delayed prolonged   D. Secretion of exogenous mediators
       leakage   by endothelial cells
                                       E. Surrounding tissue and
                                          endothelium damaged

14 Which *one* of the following is *not* an endogenous mediator of increased vascular
    permeability?
    A. Angiotensin
    B. C3a and C5a
    C. 5-hydroxytryptamine
    D. Kallikrein
    E. Prostaglandin E_2

10   **a = E**   The commonest cause of cardiogenic shock is myocardial infarction; but rupture of a heart valve, cardiac tamponade or arrythmia can cause it.

     b = A   Hypovolaemic shock usually results from trauma – severe haemorrhage or burns being the usual cause. In extensive burns there is considerable exudation of plasma resulting in hypovolaemia.

     c = B   Septic shock occurs in patients with septicaemia or extensive localised infections, e.g. peritonitis; it may complicate gastrointestinal, urogenital or biliary surgery and can occur in immunosuppressed patients.
         The shock of pancreatitis (D) is probably chemical in nature, while that of incompatible blood transfusion (C) is the result of an immunologically-mediated reaction.

11   **B**   In the acute inflammatory response the injury results in an initial contraction of arterioles (A) followed rapidly by arteriolar and venular dilatation (C) in the process of active hyperaemia; as a result of this hyperaemia the inflammatory exudate is formed (E) and is responsible for swelling and pain; the microcirculation remains engorged, but blood flow slows down (B) with associated emigration of leucocytes (D).

12   **B**   There is experimental evidence that gaps appear between vascular endothelial cells during acute inflammation caused by injury and chemical mediators. These gaps are temporary. Micropinocytotic vesicles (A) do transfer material across cells but are not increased in inflammation.

13   **a = E**   This occurs in more severe injury in which vascular damage may be so great as to cause thrombosis and even infarction of the tissues.

     b = B   In the experimental models only, venular leakage occurs in this phase; this suggests endogenous mediator activity, and histamine is usually involved.

     c = C   Both venules and capillaries leak in this phase, but leakage is confined to the zone of injury suggesting that this is due to direct endothelial injury of mild degree, since necrosis is not seen.

14   **A**   Angiotensin is produced by the action of renin on angiotensinogen and is involved in the secretion of aldosterone and in pressor effects. C3a and C5a (B) are part of the complement cascade and are activated C3 and C5; they act by liberating histamine from mast cells. 5-hydroxytryptamine (C) or serotonin causes increased vascular permeability in rodents but not in man. Kallikrein (D) is produced by activation of Hageman factor producing a prekallikrein activator that converts prekallikrein to kallikrein. Prostaglandin E_2 (E) is secreted by polymorphs, which are phagocytically active, it does not cause increased permeability itself but potentiates the activity of other factors.

15 Which *one* of the following is *not* a useful effect of acute inflammation?
    A. Dilution of toxins
    B. Formation of fibrin
    C. Phagocytosis
    D. Stimulation of the immune response
    E. Swelling of tissues

16 Which *one* of the following is *not* an acceptable characteristic of a granuloma?
    A. Composed of altered macrophages
    B. Composed of fused macrophages (giant cells)
    C. Composed of epithelioid cells
    D. Composed of a mixture of chronic inflammatory cells
    E. Composed of polymorphonuclear leucocytes, cellular
        debris and fibrin

17 From the list on the right choose the most suitable association for each of the
    types of collagen listed on the left.
    a. Type I collagen   A. Basement membrane
    b. Type II collagen   B. Cartilage
    c. Type III collagen   C. Dermis
                               D. Embryonic dermis
                               E. Synovial membrane

18 If the following events in the healing of an open wound were in their most
    probable order which would come *fourth*?
    A. Emigration of polymorphonuclear leucocytes and macrophages
    B. Epithelial proliferation
    C. Myofibroblast contraction
    D. Orientation of fibroblasts parallel to capillary buds
    E. Proliferation of new capillaries from the base of the wound

19 Which *one* of the following does *not* impair wound healing?
    A. Deficiency of vitamin C
    B. Deficiency of zinc
    C. Excess of adrenal glucocorticoid hormones
    D. Good vascular supply
    E. Tissue hypoxia

15   **E**   Tissue swelling may result in obstruction of a vital passageway, e.g. larynx, or may cause ischaemic necrosis within an enclosed space, e.g. testis.

The others are all useful *but* some people may have an inappropriate immune response and may therefore develop a pathological condition as part of their physiological response, e.g. asthmatics. There is also a rare condition in which a deficiency of a complement activation controlling factor (C1-inhibitor) allows complement activation to occur (angio-neurotic oedema).

16   **E**   This is a description of pus as would be found in an abscess. Polymorphonuclear leucocytes and nuclear debris can be found in a true granuloma if there is a focus of suppuration.

The definition of 'granuloma' is controversial; it may be used to mean a chronic inflammatory lesion forming a tissue mass or it may be restricted to a lesion composed of macrophages or altered macrophages (epithelioid cells).

17   **a = C**   Type I collagen is the major interstitial collagen, found in dermis, bone, cornea and tendon.

      b = B   Type II collagen is found in cartilage, intervertebral disc and vitreous body.

      c = A   Type III collagen is found in basement membrane; it does not form fibrils.

Seven different types of collagen are described: Types I and III are the most important for healing.

18   **D**   In a wound healing by second intention (either an open wound or ulcer with loss of tissue, or an infected wound) there is emigration of polymorphonuclear leucocytes, macrophages from the vessels (A) initially with the presence of more abundant fibrinous exudate. Epithelial proliferation (B) is the first sign of healing followed by the proliferation of capillary buds (E) forming granulation tissue with the associated proliferating fibroblasts (D). The fibroblast orientation later becomes parallel to the epithelial surface and contractility of these myofibroblasts (C) helps to reduce the area of the open wound. Scar tissue is usually more prominent than in first intention healing.

19   **D**   Wounds in areas of poor vascularity (e.g. the skin of the shin) heal very slowly compared with wounds of the face and scalp. Tissue hypoxia following severe injury results in poor healing (E). Vitamin C and zinc (A,B) are essential for the repair of ground substances and collagen. Excessive glucocorticoids (C) are associated with poor healing, and this may be seen in patients on long-term steroid therapy.

20 Which of the following events occurs *fourth* in sequence after fracture of a
    typical long bone?
    A. Capillary proliferation from viable marrow
    B. Increased osteoclastic resorption
    C. Lamellar bone replaces woven bone
    D. Ossification of the persistent fibrin clot
    E. Periosteal proliferation around the fractured bone ends

21 For each of the cells involved in the immune response listed on the left select
    the most appropriate function from the list on the right.
    a. Accessory cell   A. Antigen-stimulated lymphocyte
    b. Effector lymphocyte   that is proliferating
    c. Natural killer cell   B. Bone marrow-derived lymphocyte
                                        C. Fully differentiated product
                                           of an antigen-stimulated
                                           lymphoblast
                                        D. Kills target cells without prior
                                           sensitisation or antigen
                                           specificity
                                        E. Non-lymphoid cell which
                                           modulates immune responses

22 For each of the features of a lymph node listed on the left select the most
    appropriate association from the list on the right.
    a. Expansion of the   A. Macrophages predominate
       deep cortex   B. Plasma cells predominate
    b. Primary lymphoid   C. Region of T-cell response
       follicles   D. Superficial cortex of
    c. Production of   stimulated lymph node
       germinal centres   E. Superficial cortex of
                                           unstimulated lymph node

23 For each of the features of the immunoglobulin molecule listed on the left select
    the most appropriate association from the list on the right.
    a. Fab fragment   A. C-terminal region
    b. Fc fragment   B. Consists of heavy chains only
    c. F(ab^1)$_2$ fragment   C. Consists of the light chain and
                                           part of the heavy chain
                                        D. Consists of light chains only
                                        E. Pepsin digestion product

20   **D**   Following fracture of a long bone, provisional callus is formed by the proliferation of periosteal inner layer (E) that forms a cuff of bone trabeculae, which produces the external callus; medullary cavity reaction (A) results in organisation of the fibrin clot with production of woven bone in the marrow spaces; cortical reaction (B) results in increased osteoclastic resorption. The external callus unites the fragments externally, but not the bone ends that are joined by the fibrin clot and debris, which in turn are ossified by osteogenic cells from the medullary cavity and periosteal callus (D). The final step is remodelling of the bone (C) with formation of lamellar bone and resorption of the external callus, and eventually medullary callus.

21 **a = E**   Many of these cells resemble mononuclear phagocytes.
They are usually Ia positive, and are essential for T-helper cell activity.

    b = C   These are the functional cells of the immune response, e.g. plasma cells.

    c = D   These cells have large intracytoplasmic granules (large granular lymphocytes) that aid identification.
Activated lymphocytes (A) take an active part in the immune response. B-lymphocytes are bone marrow-derived (B) and differentiate into antibody-producing plasma cells.

22 **a = C**   The deep (or para) cortex is the T-lymphocytic zone of the lymph node and enlarges during antigenic stimulus resulting in cell-mediated resonse.

    b = E   In the unstimulated lymph node there are localised aggregates of lymphocytes in the superficial cortex.

    c = D   Following antigenic stimulation resulting in antibody production (humoral) the primary follicles enlarge to become germinal centres where B-lymphocytes proliferate.
During the humoral response plasma cells are produced and these may be seen in the cortex deep to the germinal centres and in the medullary cords (B).
Macrophages are present lining the sinuses (A) and may become very prominent (sinus histiocytosis).

23 **a = C**   Papain digestion of monomeric immunoglobulin results in the production of two antibody binding fragments (Fab) that consist of light chains plus part of the heavy chain.

    b = A   Papain digestion of monomeric immunoglobulin results in the production of a fragment consisting of the C-terminal ends of the heavy chains linked together (Fc)

    c = E   Pepsin digestion splits the immunoglobulin molecule to produce a fragment consisting of two Fab fragments united by a portion of the Fc fragment $(F(ab^1)_2)$.

24 For each class of immunoglobulin listed on the left select the most appropriate
    association from the list on the right.
    a. IgG   A. J-chain
    b. IgM   B. Lymphocyte surface antigen
    c. Dimeric IgA   receptor
                                          C. Mast cell degranulation
                                          D. Primary antibody response
                                          E. Secondary antibody response

25 For each type of T-lymphocyte listed on the left select the most appropriate
    description from the list on the right.
    a. Cytotoxic T-cell   A. Antigen specific lysis by direct
    b. Delayed type   cell to cell contact
       hypersensitivity   B. Assists antibody production
       T-cell   C. Class II MHC positive cell
    c. Helper T-cell   D. CD3-negative cell
                                          E. Release of cytokines

26 If the following features of *the atopic reaction* were placed in their correct order
    which would come *fourth*?
    A. Antigen absorbed for the second time
    B. Degranulation of mast cells
    C. Inhalation of pollen
    D. Mast cell binding by Fc component of IgE
    E. Production of IgE

27 For each of the hypersensitivity reactions listed on the left select the most
    appropriate association from the conditions on the right.
    a. Antibody dependent   A. Asthma
       cytotoxicity   B. Auto-immune haemolytic anaemia
    b. Arthus reaction   C. Extrinsic allergic alveolitis
    c. Delayed   D. Infantile eczema
       hypersensitivity   E. Tuberculoid leprosy
       reaction

28 Which *one* of the following is *not* an organ specific autoimmune disease?
    A. Addison's disease
    B. Juvenile diabetes mellitus
    C. Hashimoto's thyroiditis
    D. Pernicious anaemia
    E. Rheumatoid arthritis

24 **a = E**   Following injection of antigen into an animal not
    b = D   previously exposed to that antigen there is a transient appearance
              in the blood of a small quantity of specific IgM in about 7 days
              (primary antibody response); re-injection of the antigen results
              in production of IgG in large amounts within 4 days (secondary
              antibody response).

    c = A   Secretory IgA is a dimer, i.e. 2 molecules linked together by a
              polypeptide, J-chain. (IgM is also produced as a pentamer, the 5
              IgM molecules being linked by 1 J-chain and 4 disulphide bonds).
              Mast cell degranulation (C) is a property of IgE. Lymphocyte surface
              antigen receptor (B) is a property of IgD.

25 **a = A**   Cytotoxic T-cells are fully differentiated antigen specific T-cells
              which destroy cells by direct cell to cell contact. They are MHC I
              restricted, CD8+ cells.

    b = E   DTH cells are class II MHC restricted, CD4+ T cells which release
              cytokines such as interferon-γ.

    c = B   Helper T-cells are one of two groups of regulatory T-cells.
              Antigen presenting cells are MHC II positive and internalise and
              process complex antigens (C).
              Natural killer (NK) cells possess some T-cell markers (CD2, CD8) but
              are CD3 negative (D) and are probably a third lymphocyte lineage.

26 **A**   Atopy (anaphylactic, immediate or type 1 hypersensitivity) occurs
              when IgE binds to mast cells and causes degranulation; antigen is
              absorbed (C) and the immune response produces specific IgE (E),
              which binds by its Fc component to Fc_E-receptors on mast cells
              (D); subsequent exposure to antigen (A) results in antigen trapping
              by the IgE Fab components on the mast cells with subsequent
              degranulation (B) and activation of phospholipase A_2 and C.

27 **a = B**   Cytotoxic antibody (type 2) reactions are mediated by antibody
              which combines with cell surface antigenic determinants usually
              causing lysis. Auto-immune haemolytic anaemia, idiopathic
              thrombocytopenic purpura are examples.

    b = C   Immune complex, Arthus type (localised type 3) reaction is the basis
              of extrinsic allergic alveolitis (farmer's lung), which is a reaction to
              bacterial spores growing on mouldy hay.

    c = E   Delayed hypersensitivity (type 4) reactions are mediated by primed
              T-lymphocytes; tuberculoid leprosy, tuberculosis and contact
              dermatitis are examples. Asthma and infantile eczema are examples
              of atopy (type 1).

28 **A.**   Rheumatoid arthritis is one of the group of connective tissue
              diseases with evidence of an auto-immune pathogenesis.
              Rheumatoid factor consists of IgM antibodies to altered IgG,
              which is auto-antigenic.

29 For each of the types of immune deficiency state listed on the left select the most appropriate defect from the list on the right.
    a. Di George syndrome   A. Defective B-cell function
    b. Infantile X-linked   B. Defective B- and T-cell
       agammaglobulinaemia   function
    c. Severe combined   C. Defective T-cell function
       immunodeficiency   D. Defective platelets
                                           E. Defective vessels

30 For each of the biochemical defects listed on the left select the most appropriate association from the list of diseases on the right.
    a. C1 inhibitor   A. Autosomal recessive Chronic
       deficiency   Granulomatous Disease (CGD)
    b. Cytochrome b-245   B. Chediak-Higashi syndrome
       deficiency   C. Hereditary angio-oedema
    c. NK cell function   D. Myeloperoxidase deficiency
       absent   syndrome
                                           E. X-linked CGD

31 Which *one* of the following is *not* a feature of amyloid?
    A. Extracellular fibrillar material
    B. Filaments of 7.5–10 nm diameter
    C. Intracellular protein
    D. Present initially in the walls of small blood vessels
    E. Shows red–green birefringence when stained with Congo Red

32 For each of the types of amyloid listed on the left select the most appropriate association from the list on the right.
    a. AA amyloid   A. Bronchopneumonia
    b. AL amyloid   B. Depression of T-cell function
    c. ASc protein amyloid   C. Elderly patients
                                           D. Multiple myeloma
                                           E. Rheumatoid arthritis

33 For each of the types of Glycogen Storage Disorder (GSD) listed on the left select the most appropriate defect from the list on the right.
    a. GSD IA (von Gierke's   A. Alpha-1,4-glucan-6-glycosyl
       disease)   transferase deficiency
    b. GSD II (Pompe's   B. Alpha-glucose-1,4-glucosidase
       disease)   deficiency
    c. GSD III   C. Amylo-1 6-glucosidase
                                              deficiency
                                           D. Glucose-6-phosphatase deficiency
                                           E. Muscle phosphorylase deficiency

34 Which *one* of the following is *not* a mucopolysaccharidosis?
    A. Fabry's disease
    B. Hunter's syndrome
    C. Hurler's syndrome
    D. Morquio's syndrome
    E. Sanfilippo's syndrome

29 **a = C** There is almost complete failure of development of the thymus and parathyroids from the 3rd and 4th branchial arches.

    b = A This selective B-cell defect (Bruton type) results in failure to produce immunoglobulins.

    c = B This combined type (Swiss type) of agammaglobulinaemia has failure of development of both thymus-dependent and -independent systems.
Platelets are abnormal (D) in the rare Wiskott–Aldrich syndrome in which T-cell function, IgM and IgA are also abnormal. Abnormal vessels (E) are a feature of ataxia telangiectasia in which there is abnormal cell-mediated immunity and low IgA and IgE.

30 **a = C** C1 inhibitor deficiency results in subcutaneous and submucosal oedema due to uncontrolled C1 activation.

    b = E Cytochrome b-245 deficiency is seen in the X-linked form of CGD, but not in the autosomal recessive form (A) where a phosphorylation reaction substrate is absent.

    c = B NK cell function is absent and neutrophils contain giant (non-functioning) granules.
Patients with myeloperoxidase deficiency (D) do not make hypochlorous acid and are susceptible to candidiasis.

31   **C** Amyloid is an extracellular substance (A) consisting of fibrillar material with a characteristic ultrastructural appearance (B). It is seen initially in the walls of small blood vessels (D) in relation to the basement membrane. The most specific histological reaction is the red–green birefringence seen with Congo Red and polarised light microscopy (E).

32 **a = E** Amyloid of this type is seen in chronic infections (tuberculosis, syphilis, osteomyelitis) as well as in patients with rheumatoid arthritis.

    b = D 15% of patients with multiple myeloma have amyloid of this type derived from immunoglobulin light chains produced by the neoplastic cells.

    c = C This type is seen in elderly patients with generalised senile amyloidosis; ASc I protein is seen in senile cardiac amyloidosis.
Bronchopneumonia (A) is an acute infection and is not associated with amyloid; bronchiectasis is a chronic lung condition often complicated by amyloid.

33 **a = D** Presents in infancy with massive hepatomegaly and hypoglycaemia. Hepatocytes contain excess glycogen.

    b = B Deficiency of acid maltase results in glycogen storage in heart, skeletal muscle and liver. Cardiac failure in infancy.

    c = C Deficiency of debranching enzyme. Less severe than type I. Diagnosed by detecting excess glycogen in erythrocytes.
Branching enzyme deficiency (A) is very rare and causes infantile hepatic cirrhosis. McArdle's disease (E) causes myopathy.

34   **A** Fabry's disease is an X-linked sphingolypidosis in which glycophospholipids are deposited as crystals with a typical zebra stripe appearance on electron microscopy. The others are all mucopolysaccharidoses in which there is intracellular deposition and urinary excretion of glycosaminoglycans. Hurler's (C) is also known as 'gargoylism'.

35 For each of the types of porphyria listed on the left select the most appropriate
    association from the list on the left.
    a. Acute intermittent   A. Abdominal pain and neuropathy
    b. Erythropoietic   B. Abdominal pain and
        protoporphyria   photosensitivity
    c. Porphyria cutanea   C. Anaemia in infancy
        tarda.   D. Dermatosis and hepatic cirrhosis
                                        E. Photosensitivity and hepatic
                                            haemosiderosis

36 For each of the features of conditions listed on the left select the most
    appropriate association from the list on the right.
    a. Bacteraemia   A. Due to bacterial endotoxins
    b. Pyaemia   B. Fragment of septic thrombus
    c. Septicaemia   C. End result of viral infection
                                        D. May be the result of vigorous
                                            teeth brushing
                                        E. Multiplication of bacteria in
                                            the blood

37 Which *one* of the following is the best definition of gangrene?
    A. Digestion of dead tissue by saprophytic bacteria
    B. Digestion of living tissue by saprophytic bacteria
    C. Gas production in dead tissue
    D. Necrosis of tissue caused by bacterial toxins
    E. Necrosis of tissue caused by ischaemia

38 The pathogenicity of the tubercle bacillus is due to which *one* of the following?
    A. Ability to multiply within macrophages
    B. Delayed hypersensitivity reaction against the bacteria
    C. Direct toxic effect on host cells
    D. Effective antibody response
    E. Necrosis caused by expanding granulomas

39 For each of the features of tuberculous infection listed on the left select the
    most appropriate association from the list on the right.
    a. Cold abscess   A. Lesion in the lung
    b. Miliary tubercles   B. Lesion in lung and hilar lymph
    c. Primary complex   nodes
                                        C. Scar tissue with calcification
                                        D. Small white lesions in the
                                            liver, spleen and kidney
                                        E. Soft white mass of caseous pus

35 **a = A**   Latent in 85% of affected individuals; usually precipitated by drugs or alcohol.
    b = D   Presents in childhood; may also develop gallstones.
    c = E   Most common type.
            Congenital erythropoietic porphyria presents with severe skin disease and anaemia in infancy (C).
            Variegate porphyria is similar to acute intermittent porphyria, but with photosensitivity (B)

36 **a = D**   Bacteraemia is the presence of small numbers of bacteria in the blood; this can occur in normal individuals, e.g. after teeth brushing (NB this may be important in patients with valvular heart disease).
    b = B   Pyaemia (pus in the blood) is the result of localised pyogenic infection damaging vascular endothelium and producing infected thrombus which breaks down.
    c = E   Septicaemia is the presence and multiplication of organisms in the blood stream; this is the most serious type.
            Bacterial exotoxins (A) are produced by living bacteria. None of these is an end result of viral infection (C) since are all are caused by bacteria.

37 **A**   In gangrene, tissue which is dead is digested by bacteria which are incapable of invading and multiplying in living tissue (saprophytes).
            Gas production (C) may be present in some forms of gangrene, particularly when caused by the anaerobic *Clostridia*. Necrosis of tissue is an essential prerequisite for gangrene, but it may be caused by ischaemia (E), i.e secondary gangrene, or by bacterial toxins (D), i.e. primary gangrene.

38 **B**   Mycobacteria stimulate a specific T-cell response of cell-mediated immunity; while this is effective in reducing the infection the delayed hypersensitivity reaction also damages the tissues. The tubercle bacilli have no demonstrable direct toxic action (C) and can survive within macrophages (A). This may account for latent infections and reactivation of tuberculosis.
            There is no significant humoral response to tubercle bacilli (D). Necrosis occurs in tuberculosis, but it is usually within the granuloma (E).

39 **a = E**   Caseous material may liquefy following invasion by polymorphs to produce tuberculous pus; this occurs in kidneys and bones and may extend into soft tissues.
    b = D   Spread by the blood stream occurs in miliary tuberculosis and organs affected contain multiple small (1–2 mm) white nodules (miliary tubercles) which undergo caseous necrosis.
    c = B   Initial infection produces the primary lesion, e.g. in the lung (A), which remains small, but bacteria spread to the regional lymph nodes to form the primary complex of primary lesion plus involved regional nodes. Scar tissue with calcification (C) is a common result of healing of tuberculosis.

40 For each of the features of syphilis listed on the left select the most appropriate
    association from the list on the right.
    a. Primary sore   A. Degeneration of posterior
    b. Secondary lesions   columns of spinal cord
    c. Tertiary lesions   B. Destruction of the nasal bones
                                       C. Miliary gummas
                                       D. Rash on the soles of the feet
                                       E. Pale brown nodules on the penis

41 Sort the following stages in viral infection into order and indicate which comes
    fourth in the sequence.
    A. Adsorption of virus to cell surface
    B. Assembly of virion
    C. Entry of virion into cell
    D. Transcription of virus mRNA
    E. Release of virion

42 Which *one* of the following is *not* a feature of interferons?
    A. Aid resistance to virus infections
    B. Encoded by genes of the host cell genome
    C. Released from cells in response to virus infections
    D. Species-specific cellular protein
    E. Virus-specific antiviral effect

43 For each of the disease states listed on the left select the most appropriate
    cause from the list on the right.
    a. Cancer cachexia   A. End-organ resistance to vitamin D
    b. Kwashiorkor   B. Sudden weaning onto a high-
    c. Wernicke–Korsakoff   carbohydrate, low-protein diet
       syndrome   C. TNF-α
                                       D. Thiamine deficiency
                                       E. Zinc deficiency

44 From the list on the right select the most appropriate definition for each of the
    terms on the left.
    a. Anaplasia   A. Complete loss of resemblance to
    b. Differentiation   the tissue of origin
    c. Dysplasia   B. Degree of resemblance to the
                                          tissue of origin
                                       C. Describes rate of growth of
                                          tumour tissue
                                       D. Partial loss of resemblance to
                                          the tissue of origin
                                       E. Tissue of origin

45 For which *one* of the following tumours is there a definite genetic basis in a
    proportion of cases?
    A. Bronchial carcinoma
    B. Cervical carcinoma
    C. Colonic carcinoma
    D. Endometrial carcinoma
    E. Vaginal carcinoma

40   **a = E**   The primary sore occurs after an incubation period of 3–4 weeks
                during which period *Treponema pallidum* is spreading in the blood.
     b = D   The secondary lesions occur 2–3 months after infection and are
                characterised by skin rashes, alopecia and general malaise.
     c = B   The typical lesions of the tertiary phase occur many years after
                infection and cause necrosis of internal organs. The gumma is a
                necrotic granuloma.
                Tabes dorsalis (A) occurs in the late quaternary phase of neuro-
                syphilis. Miliary gummas (C) are present in congenital syphilis.

41   **B**   The virion is adsorbed onto the cell surface (A) and then enters the
                cell where uncoating takes place (C). Transcription of viral RNA
                allows production of viral genomic material by the cell (D). The virion
                is then assembled (B) and released (E).

42   **E**   The production of interferons is induced in the host cells by the
                virus; the interferons are not specific, but are an important host
                defence mechanism against virus infection. They act by inhibiting
                the translation of viral mRNA by uninfected host cells.

43   **a = C**   TNF-α (cachectin) inhibits lipoprotein lipase and may cause loss of
                fat in cancer patients.
     b = B   This is the commonest cause of protein-energy malnutrition
                worldwide.
     c = D   Vitamin B_1 deficiency causes polyneuropathy (dry beriberi), cardiac
                failure (wet beriberi), and the Wernicke–Korsakoff syndrome,
                which is seen in alcoholics. There is atrophy of the mamillary
                bodies.
                End-organ resistance to Vitamin D occurs in type II vitamin D-
                dependent rickets (A); zinc deficiency (E) affects the gonads, wound
                healing, the skin and night vision.

44   **a = A**   Complete loss of resemblance to tissue of origin is a feature of
                malignant tumours.
     b = B   The degree of resemblance of a tumour to its tissue of origin:
                well-differentiated tumours closely resemble their tissue of origin,
                poorly differentiated tumours show little resemblance.
     c = D   Partial loss of resemblance to the tissue of origin is a feature of
                many pre-malignant conditions and some benign tumours.
                There is no specific term for the rate of growth of tumour tissue (C);
                the mitotic rate of a tumour gives some idea of tumour growth. The
                tissue of origin (E) is known as the histogenesis of the tumour.

45   **C**   *Polyposis (adenomatosis) coli* has a Mendelian dominant in-
                heritance, half the members of the family developing colonic
                polyps with resultant colonic cancers in early adult life. A tumour
                susceptibility gene is also present in 20% of the population.
                Some families have similar tumours occurring in siblings in several
                generations (A). Vaginal clear cell carcinoma (E) may develop in
                teenage girls whose mothers took diethyl stilboestrol in pregnancy.

46 Which *one* of the following is *not* associated with EB virus infection?
    A. Burkitt's lymphoma
    B. Carcinoma of the cervix uteri
    C. Infectious mononucleosis
    D. Nasopharyngeal carcinoma
    E. No clinical symptoms

47 For each of the types of neoplasm listed on the left select the most appropriate
    definition from the list on the right.
    a. Adenoma   A. Benign connective tissue tumour
    b. Carcinoma   B. Benign epithelial tumour derived
    c. Papilloma   from glandular tissue
                             C. Benign epithelial tumour derived
                                from a surface
                             D. Malignant connective tissue
                                tumour
                             E. Malignant epithelial tumour

48 For each of the types of tumour listed on the left select the most appropriate
    description from the list on the right.
    a. Leiomyoma   A. Benign tumour of adipose tissue
    b. Lipoma   B. Benign tumour of smooth muscle
    c. Teratoma   C. Cystic tumour of ovary
                             D. Glial tumour
                             E. Vascular tumour on finger

49 For each of the cell compartments listed on the left select the most appropriate
    description from the list on the right.
    a. Amplification   A. Cells are involved in lineage
       compartment   generation
    b. Stem cell   B. Cells are capable of
       compartment   differentiation but not
    c. Terminal   division
       differentiation   C. Cells are capable of self
       compartment   renewal and lineage generation
                             D. Cells are capable of division
                                but not differentiation
                             E. Cells are capable of self
                                renewal only

50 Which *one* of the following is *not* a non-metastatic effect of a lung cancer?
    A. Cushingoid state
    B. Dermatomyositis
    C. Raised intracranial pressure
    D. Sensory neuropathy
    E. Tumour cachexia

46	**B**	Carcinoma of the uterine cervix is associated with infection by human papilloma virus (HPV). Burkitt's lymphoma occurs when EB virus infects B-lymphocytes and causes translocation of c-*myc* proto-oncogene from chromosome 8q24 to 14q32, which is the heavy chain locus. EB infection is ubiquitous and is responsible for infectious mononucleosis (C), nasopharyngeal carcinoma (D) and is often subclinical (E).

47	**a** = **B**	These occur more commonly in endocrine than exocrine tissues and often retain secretory activity.
	b = **E**	This is a generic term that may be more fully described by prefixes such as 'adeno-', 'squamous-'.
	c = **C**	These are common tumours in the breast ducts, and may be found in the urinary tract. Some benign tumours of the intestine have been called papillomas but they are really adenomas.

48	**a** = **B**	The leiomyoma is found in the uterus where it is the commonest tumour type.
	b = **A**	These are very common subcutaneous tumours.
	c = **C**	The benign dermoid cyst of the ovary is a cystic teratoma; teratomas in the male are invariably malignant. Glial tumours (D) are malignant neuroectodermal tumours. A glomangioma is derived from the glomus body which controls blood flow and temperature in the extremities.

49	**a** = **A**	The transit or amplification compartment contains cells that are involved in the production of families of mature cells (lineage generation) by division and differentiation of precursors.
	b = **C**	Cells capable of both self renewal and lineage generation are called stem cells.
	c = **B**	Cells in which division has ceased may still differentiate, but they ultimately die.

50	**C**	Raised intracranial pressure could be due to a primary intracranial tumour or a secondary tumour. Cushingoid state is the result of secretion of ACTH by the tumour (A); dermatomyositis (B) and sensory neuropathy (D) are unexplained effects. Tumour cachexia (E) is the result of secretion of TNF and/or interleukin 1 by macrophages within the tumour.

51 For each of the causes of resistance to cancer therapy listed on the left select the most appropriate cause from the list on the right.
    a. Amplification of   A. Failure to get total kill by
       gene coding for   radiotherapy
       dihydrofolate   B. Resistance to chemotherapeutic
       reductase   agents
    b. Cells in G_0 phase   C. Resistance to etoposides
    c. P170 glycoprotein   D. Resistance to methotrexate
                                     E. Resistance to tamoxifen

52 For each of the human oncogene types listed on the left select the most appropriate association from the list on the right.
    a. Cellular oncogene   A. Ability to create the
    b. Proto-oncogene   transformed phenotype
    c. Viral oncogene   B. Expression prevents neoplasia
                                     C. Non-transforming genes
                                     D. Retrovirus transforming genes
                                     E. Viral genome integration

53 For each of the types of drug reaction on the left select the most appropriate association from the list on the right.
    a. Irreversible   A. Full recovery expected
    b. Type A   B. Immunologically determined
    c. Type B   mechanism
                                     C. Occurs in 100% of patients
                                        exposed to the drug
                                     D. Recovery occurs after formation
                                        of a new enzyme or receptor
                                     E. Results from a known
                                        pharmacological property of the
                                        drug

54 For each of the drugs listed on the left select the most appropriate reaction from the list on the right.
    a. Chlorpromazine   A. Chronic hepatitis
    b. Methyldopa   B. Liver cell adenoma
    c. Phenytoin   C. Microvesicular steatosis
                                     D. Mixed hepatitic/cholestatic
                                        reaction
                                     E. Veno-occlusive disease

55 For each of the forms of atheroma listed on the left select the most appropriate association from the list on the right.
    a. Atheromatous   A. Affects vessels of less than 2 mm
       aneurysm   diameter
    b. Complicated   B. Fat in intimal smooth muscle
       atheroma   cells
    c. Early atheromatous   C. Mucoid degeneration of the
       lesion   media
                                     D. Thinning of the media with loss
                                        of elasticity
                                     E. Ulceration of the plaque with
                                        mural thrombus formation

51   **a = D**   Methotrexate inhibits dihydrofolate reductase.

      b = A   Many tumour cells, particularly in areas of hypoxia, are in G_0 phase. Proliferating cells are killed by radiotherapy, and the G_0 cells then enter the proliferation cycle as a new generation of growing tumour cells.

      c = B   P170 glycoprotein is a membrane export system which is coded for by a gene known as *mdr* (multiple drug resistance). It is present in many colonic cancers.

             The etoposides (C) inhibit topoisomerase 2, which often mutates in tumour cells confering drug resistance. Tumours without oestrogen receptors are resistant to tamoxifen (E).

52   **a = A**   Altered version of the normal gene which regulates cell growth; *c-oncs* are able to transform cells.

      b = C   These are the normal genes of which *c-oncs* are the abnormal form.

      c = D   Retrovirus transforming genes are viral oncogenes (*v-onc*).

             Oncosuppressor genes (B) appear to prevent neoplasia.

             If these genes are inactivated this may predispose to tumour development.

             There is no evidence for viral genomic integration in any human tumours, but there are animal examples (E).

53   **a = D**   Irreversible drug reactions result in cell death or permanent damage to cellular function. Recovery may occur if an adaptive response takes place or undamaged cells multiply.

      b = E   These are dose-dependent predictable reactions.

      c = B   These are unpredictable reactions often mediated by an immunological response or due to a genetically determined host defect.

             Full recovery (A) is expected in reversible (functional) reactions. No drug would be licensed if there was a 100% incidence of reactions (C).

54   **a = D**   Chlorpromazine gives a cholestatic reaction.

      b = A   Methyldopa is the classical example of a drug-induced hepatitis.

      c = C   The anticonvulsant phenytoin results in fatty change.

             Veno-occlusive disease (E) is caused by pyrrolizidine alkaloids. Liver cell adenomas (B) may occur with contraceptive steroids.

55   **a = D**   Thinning of the media with extension of plaque into it results in loss of elasticity and may allow an aneurysm to form; this usually occurs in the lower abdominal aorta.

      b = E   Plaques showing ulceration, thrombosis and calcification represent severe disease.

      c = B   The earliest changes are fat in intimal smooth muscle cells and macrophages.

             Erdheim's medial degeneration is a mucoid change (C), which may cause dissecting aneurysm. Atheroma usually affects vessels of more than 2 mm diameter (A).

56   Which *one* of the following is *not* a predisposing factor for atheroma?
     A. Cigarette smoking
     B. High level of serum high-density lipoprotein (HDL)
     C. High level of serum low-density lipoprotein (LDL)
     D. Male sex
     E. Systemic hypertension

57   For each of the types of systemic hypertension listed on the left select the most
     appropriate association from the list on the right.

     a. Chronic benign   A. Hyaline arteriolosclerosis
        essential   B. Hyaline arteriolosclerosis with
        hypertension in a   fibrinoid necrosis
        small vessel   C. Hypertrophy of medial muscle and
     b. Early benign   elastic
        essential   D. Medial calcification
        hypertension   E. Medial and intimal necrosis of a
     c. Malignant   segment of arterial wall
        hypertension

58   Which *one* of the following is *not* involved in the aetiology of systemic
     hypertension.
     A. Arteriolosclerosis
     B. Chronic glomerulonephritis
     C. Conn's syndrome
     D. Phaeochromocytoma
     E. Raised sodium intake

59   From the list of diseases on the left select the most appropriate histological
     description from the list on the left.

     a. Infiltration of   A. Buerger's disease
        aortic adventitia   B. Giant cell (temporal) arteritis
        with plasma cells   C. Raynaud's disease
        and lymphocytes   D. Rheumatic arteritis
     b. Peri-arteritis and   E. Syphilitic aortitis
        endarteritis of the
        aortic vasa vasorum
     c. Thrombotic occlusion
        of short lengths of
        arteries and veins
        of limbs

60   If the following events were placed in chronological order which would come
     fourth?
     A. Left ventricular hypertrophy
     B. Occlusion of right coronary artery
     C. Pyelonephritis
     D. Rupture of left ventricle
     E. Systemic hypertension

56   **B**   High levels of serum HDL are associated with decreased risk of ischaemic heart disease; HDL may act as a clearance mechanism for cellular cholesterol.
High serum LDL is the major risk factor of atheroma (C).

57 **a = A** Hyaline arteriolosclerosis is the lesion of chronic benign essential hypertension in a small vessel in which there is medial thickening plus intimal thickening, which may narrow the lumen.

    b = C The early features of benign essential hypertension involve hypertrophy of medial muscle and elastic; larger vessels often dilate.

    c = B In malignant hypertension there is necrosis added to the features of benign hypertension, with permeation of the vessel wall by plasma and fibrin.
Medial calcification (D) is dystrophic calcification of the larger vessels of the lower limbs in elderly people (Mönckeberg's sclerosis). Polyarteritis nodosa has the features described in (E).

58   **A**   Arteriolosclerosis is the result of hypertension.
Renal hypertension is usually the result of chronic glomerulonephritis (B) or chronic pyelonephritis.
Conn's syndrome (primary hyperaldosteronism) is due to an adrenal tumour secreting aldosterone (C).
Phaeochromocytomas (D) secrete catecholamines.
Population studies have shown hypertension to correlate well with high average salt intake (E).

59 **a = D** Lesions similar to those seen in the heart in rheumatic fever can be found in the walls of larger vessels.

    b = E The arteritic lesion of syphilis involves the whole vessel wall; damage to the vasa vasorum results in damage to the aortic media with aneurysm formation, usually in the thoracic aorta.

    c = A Buerger's disease (thromboangiitis obliterans) involves both arteries and veins.
Giant cell (temporal) arteritis (B) occurs in the elderly; there is destruction of the elastic lamina with giant cell formation.
Raynaud's disease (C) is associated with abnormal spasm of digital vessels.

60   **B**   Chronic pyelonephritis (C) results in systemic hypertension (E) with left ventricular hypertrophy (A); hypertension is associated with increased risk of atheroma and thrombotic occlusion of a coronary artery (B), which causes myocardial infarction, complicated by necrosis of the left ventricular wall and eventual rupture (D).

61   Which *one* of the following is least likely to be found in a child dying of acute
     rheumatic fever?
     A. Aschoff bodies
     B. 'Bread and Butter' pericarditis
     C. History of recent sore throat
     D. Large crumbling vegetations on the mitral valve
     E. Raised antistreptolysin 0 titre (ASO titre)

62   For each of the valvular abnormalities on the left select the most appropriate
     association from the list of conditions on the right.
     a. Combined aortic   A. Carcinoid syndrome
        incompetence and   B. Congenital bicuspid valve
        mitral stenosis   C. Marfan's syndrome
     b. Mitral incompetence   D. Rheumatic endocarditis
     c. Pulmonary stenosis   E. Senile change in valve

63   Which is *fourth* in the following sequence of events?
     A. Bacteraemia
     B. Infective endocarditis
     C. Mitral stenosis
     D. Tonsillectomy
     E. Valvular vegetations

64   Which *one* of the following is an example of acyanotic congenital heart disease?
     A. Anomalous venous drainage
     B. Coarctation of the aorta
     C. Fallot's tetralogy
     D. Tricuspid atresia
     E. Truncus arteriosus

65   Which *one* of the following is *not* a histological feature of chronic bronchitis?
     A. Calcification of bronchial cartilages
     B. Goblet cell metaplasia
     C. Hypertrophy of smooth muscle
     D. Mucous gland hyperplasia
     E. Squamous metaplasia of respiratory epithelium

61   **D**   The vegetations of acute rheumatic fever are usually small nodular aggregates of fibrin and platelets along the line of apposition of the valve cusps.

Aschoff bodies (A) are pathognomonic of rheumatic carditis. Pericarditis of an exudative fibrinous type (B) is present as rheumatic fever is a pancarditis: the 'bread and butter' appearance is due to the sticky fibrinous exudate. A recent sore throat due to infection by β-haemolytic streptococci (C) is reflected in the raised ASO titre (E).

62   **a = D**   Mitral stenosis and aortic incompetence are a common result of chronic rheumatic heart disease.

      b = C   Mitral incompetence due to myxoid degeneration of the valve cusps occurs in the rare Marfan's syndrome; the 'floppy' mitral valve syndrome has similar histological features but is not associated with congenital anomalies.

      c = A   In the carcinoid syndrome metastatic carcinoid tumour is associated with release of 5-hydroxytryptamine into the systemic circulation, causing fibroblast proliferation in the valve cusps and ring.

Bicuspid aortic valve (B) is a common congenital anomaly. Senile changes in heart valves are usually related to calcification of the cusps (E).

63   **B**   Infective endocarditis usually follows bacteraemia (A) in a patient with some abnormality of the heart valves (C). This is often associated with previous rheumatic fever, although congenital anomalies are also involved.

Tonsillectomy (D) is the cause of the bacteraemia, which results in large soft crumbly vegetations on the abnormal valve cusps. (The order is C-D-A-B-E).

64   **B**   Coarctation of the aorta occurs predominantly in males and is a narrowing of the aorta between the left subclavian artery and the orifice of the ductus arteriosus. The others are all examples of cyanotic anomalies in which systemic venous blood is mixed with oxygenated blood leaving the heart; the red cell count rises, which increases the cyanosis.

65   **C**   Smooth muscle hypertrophy is seen in bronchial asthma.

The histological features of chronic bronchitis include hyperplasia of the mucous glands (D) and goblet cell metaplasia in the terminal bronchioles (B). Respiratory epithelium may undergo squamous metaplasia (E), and calcification of cartilages (A) can occur.

66   For each of the types of bronchial asthma listed on the left select the most
     appropriate association from the list on the right.
     a. Extrinsic asthma   A. Commences in childhood
     b. Intrinsic asthma   B. No allergen implicated
     c. Status asthmaticus   C. Prolonged attack with severe
                                         respiratory distress
                                      D. Right ventricular hypertrophy
                                      E. Type III hypersensitivity
                                         reaction

67   If the following were placed in chronological order which would come *fourth*?
     A. Bronchiectasis
     B. Bronchopulmonary anastomoses
     C. Congestive cardiac failure
     D. Raised pulmonary artery pressure
     E. Whooping cough

68   Which *one* of the following is least likely to result in a sustained rise in
     pulmonary artery pressure?
     A. Atrial septal defect
     B. Chronic bronchitis and emphysema
     C. Lobar pneumonia
     D. Pulmonary fibrosis
     E. Pulmonary thrombo-embolic disease

69   For each of the types of pulmonary emphysema listed on the left select the
     most appropriate association from the list on the right.
     a. Alveolar duct   A. Air in the interlobular septae
        emphysema   B. Enlargement of alveolar ducts,
     b. Bronchiolar emphysema   spaces and respiratory
     c. Panacinar emphysema   bronchioles
                                      C. Enlargement of centrilobular air
                                         spaces
                                      D. Fusiform dilatation of alveolar
                                         ducts surrounded by coal dust
                                      E. Normal respiratory bronchioles
                                         with enlarged ducts and alveoli

70   For each of the types of pneumonia listed on the left select the most
     appropriate association from the list on the right.
     a. Aspiration   A. Interstitial mononuclear cell
        pneumonia   infiltrate
     b. Bronchopneumonia   B. *Legionella pneumophila* identified
        with abscess   in lung sections
        formation   C. Spontaneous resolution on the
     c. Recently discovered   8th day
        form of lobar   D. Sputum culture yields *Klebsiella*
        pneumonia   *pneumoniae*
                                      E. Suppurative bronchopneumonia
                                         with foreign body giant cells

66   **a = A**   This usually occurs in childhood, often with a history of eczema or food allergy; there is often a detectable allergen which triggers a Type I (atopic) reaction.

     b = B   This usually develops in adults with no atopic history, although drug hypersensitivities may develop; there is an association with bronchitis.

     c = C   Status asthmaticus is a continuous attack of asthma, with severe respiratory distress that may be fatal; at autopsy the lungs are distended with air, and plugs of mucus are present in segmental bronchi.

           Right ventricular hypertrophy (D) is not usually a feature of bronchial asthma except in rare cases where alveolar hypoxia results in pulmonary hypertension.

           Type III hypersensitivity reactions occur in extrinsic allergic alveolitis (E).

67   **D**   Whooping cough in childhood (E) results in the formation of bronchiectasis (A) by pulmonary collapse and imperfect resolution of pneumonia; bronchiectasis disturbs the pulmonary haemodynamics such that bronchopulmonary anastomoses (B) are formed that result in raised pulmonary artery pressure (D); right ventricular hypertrophy with congestive cardiac failure may follow (C).

68   **C**   Lobar pneumonia is usually a short-term illness with resolution without chronic lung damage. Congenital cardiac shunts which are pre-tricuspid (A) produce pulmonary hypertension in adolescence. Chronic bronchitis and emphysema (B) and pulmonary fibrosis (D) result in damage to the vascular tree as a result of chronic hypoxia. Recurrent pulmonary thrombo-embolism (E) leads to a progressive increase in pulmonary vascular resistance.

69   **a = E**   This is the initial stage of alveolar emphysema.

     b = C   This is centrilobular emphysema (more common in male smokers) and is more serious than the other form of bronchiolar emphysema (focal dust emphysema), which occurs in coal workers.

     c = B   This is the late stage of alveolar emphysema in which the entire respiratory acinus is involved.

           In focal dust emphysema there is fusiform dilatation of the respiratory bronchioles which are surrounded by coal dust (D).

           Air in the interlobular spaces (A) is interstitial emphysema caused by rupture of the air spaces, usually as a result of overdistention or trauma.

70   **a = E**   Aspiration of gastric contents results in pneumonia with a foreign body giant cell reaction to vegetable and meat fibres.

     b = D   Klebsiellar pneumonia is characterized by mucoid destruction of the right upper lobe and progression to destructive lung disease.

     c = B   Legionnaires's disease is a recently described (1976) form of lobar pneumonia caused by an organism that contaminates the environment, particularly in air conditioning and shower water supply tanks.

           Interstitial mononuclear cell infiltration (A) is characteristic of viral pneumonia. Spontaneous resolution on the 8th day is a feature of classical pneumococcal lobar pneumonia (C).

71 Which *one* of the following compounds is *not* associated with pulmonary fibrosis or alveolar damage?
    A. Busulphan
    B. Nitrofurantoin
    C. Paraquat
    D. Penicillamine
    E. Stilboestrol

72 For each of the forms of industrial lung disease on the left select the most appropriate association from the list on the right.
    a. Asbestosis
    b. Byssinosis
    c. Caplan's syndrome

    A. Bronchoconstriction due to cotton dust
    B. Fibrosis in sub-pleural region of the lower lobes
    C. Lung lesions in miners with rheumatoid arthritis
    D. Particles of carbon in alveolar macrophages
    E. Sarcoid-like reaction in lungs

73 Which *one* of the following events comes *fourth* in chronological order?
    A. Bronchial carcinoma
    B. Cerebral metastases
    C. Raised intracranial pressure
    D. Smoking 40 cigarettes per day
    E. Squamous metaplasia of respiratory epithelium

74 For each of the tumours listed on the left select the most appropriate association from the list on the right
    a. Bronchial carcinoid
    b. Oat cell carcinoma
    c. Pleural mesothelioma

    A. Chance finding on chest X-ray
    B. Commonest at periphery of lung
    C. Mixed histological pattern
    D. Slow-growing malignant tumour
    E. Usually arises from main bronchus at hilum

75 For each of the causes of anaemia listed on the left select the most appropriate association from the list on the right.
    a. Excessive destruction of erythrocytes
    b. Excessive loss of erythrocytes
    c. Diminished production of erythrocytes with marrow hyperplasia

    A. Acholuric jaundice
    B. Deficiency of vitamin B_{12}
    C. Therapy with chloramphenicol
    D. Fibrosis of haemopoietic marrow
    E. Massive gastrointestinal haemorrhage

71   **E**   Stilboestrol is not known to cause pulmonary fibrosis.
The other compounds may all cause pulmonary fibrosis: paraquat (C), taken either accidently or intentionally, causes severe intra-alveolar fibrosis.

72   **a = B**   Asbestos exposure is associated with pleural fibrous plaques, fibrosis of the lung (asbestosis) and mesothelioma.

    b = A   This occurs after many years of exposure to cotton dust; it is indistinguishable from chronic bronchitis.

    c = C   Pneumoconiosis and rheumatoid arthritis are associated with large rounded nodules in the lung which may undergo necrosis and resemble tuberculosis or cancer.
The presence of carbon in macrophages (D) is known as anthracosis and is almost universal. The metal beryllium causes sarcoid-like reactions in lung, liver and lymph nodes (E).

73   **B**   Cigarette smoking (D) results in chronic irritation of the ciliated respiratory epithelium that undergoes squamous metaplasia (E). Bronchial carcinoma develops (A) and may metastasize (B) to the brain where it will act as a space-occupying lesion causing raised intracranial pressure (C).

74   **a = D**   The bronchial carcinoid protrudes into the bronchial lumen and invades locally. It contains neurosecretory granules.

    b = E   This type of tumour may be associated with endocrine symptoms; it usually occurs at the hilum and is derived from endocrine cells.

    c = C   Mesotheliomas often show a mixed pattern of papillary adenocarcinoma and spindle cell tumour; it is associated with previous exposure to asbestos, particularly crocidolite.
The benign adenochondroma is often a chance finding on X-ray (A); it is a hamartomatous lesion consisting of cartilage and lung tissue. Adenocarcinomas of the lung usually arise at the periphery (B) and are often associated with scar tissue.

75   **a = A**   In haemolytic anaemia there is destruction of erythrocytes with excessive production of bilirubin, which is conjugated and therefore not excreted in the urine.

    b = E   Erythrocytes are usually lost in large numbers following a large bleed; if bleeding stops there is a brisk marrow response (reticulocytosis); chronic small blood losses result in iron-deficiency anaemia.

    c = B   Pernicious anaemia is due to lack of vitamin B_{12} and folic acid, and is a megaloblastic anaemia; this is an example of a dyshaemopoietic state (as is iron-deficiency anaemia).
Idiosyncratic reactions to drugs (C) result in aplastic anaemia in which the marrow is hypocellular.
Myelofibrosis is a myeloproliferative disorder with fibrous replacement of the marrow (D) resulting in anaemia.

76 For each of the types of haemolytic anaemia listed on the left select the most
    appropriate description from the list on the right.

    a. Haemolytic disease   A. Abnormal sensitivity to cold
       of the newborn   B. Defect in haemoglobin polypeptide
    b. Hereditary   chain
       spherocytosis   C. Genetically determined red cell
    c. Microangiopathic   defect
       haemolytic anaemia   D. Red cell fragmentation
                                       E. Rhesus incompatability

77 Which *one* of the following is *not* a cause of vitamin B_{12} deficiency?
    A. Blind-loop syndrome
    B. Dietary deficiency
    C. Intrinsic factor deficiency
    D. Resection of ascending colon
    E. Resection of terminal ileum

78 For each of the types of acute leukaemia listed on the left select the most
    appropriate association from the list on the right.

    a. Acute lymphoblastic   A. Immunoglobulin heavy-chain
       leukaemia (L1)   rearrangement
    b. Acute monocytic   B. Leukaemic cells with cytoplasmic
       leukaemia (M5)   projections
    c. Undifferentiated   C. No cytochemical markers
       myeloblastic   D. Philadelphia chromosome positive
       leukaemia (M0)   E. Sodium fluoride-sensitive
                                          non-specific esterase activity

79 Gross splenomegaly is a striking feature of which *one* of the following?
    A. Acute lymphoblastic leukaemia
    B. Acute monocytic leukaemia
    C. Acute myeloblastic leukaemia
    D. Acute myelomonocytic leukaemia
    E. Chronic granulocytic leukaemia

80 For each of the types of plasma cell tumour listed on the left select the most
    appropriate association from the list on the right.

    a. Heavy-chain disease   A. Bence–Jones proteinuria
    b. Light-chain disease   B. Increased blood viscosity
    c. Macroglobulinaemia   C. Increased red cell mass
                                       D. Mediterranean lymphoma
                                       E. Solitary tumour in a long bone

81 Which *one* of the following is the commonest neoplastic cause of enlarge-
    ment of lymph nodes?
    A. Chronic lymphatic leukaemia
    B. Diffuse non-Hodgkin's lymphoma
    C. Follicular lymphoma
    D. Nodular sclerosis Hodgkin's disease
    E. Secondary carcinoma

76	**a = E**	Rhesus incompatability results in maternal iso-antibody production, which crosses the placenta and may cause haemolysis in the baby.
	b = C	This is an autosomal dominant condition in which the red cell membrane protein spectrin is deficient.
	c = D	Red cell fragmentation occurs in conditions in which small vessels are criss-crossed by strands of fibrin.

Abnormal sensitivity to cold (A) is one form of autoimmune haemolytic anaemia in which cold-agglutinins form. Defective haemoglobin synthesis (B) results in the haemoglobinopathies.

77   **D**   Vitamin B_{12} complexed with intrinsic factor (C) is absorbed in the terminal ileum, disease or resection of which will cause failure of absorption (E).

Dietary deficiency (B) can occur (usually in vegans).

Blind-loop syndrome (A) occurs when bacteria in a loop of bowel proximal to the terminal ileum take up the B_{12}-IF complex before it reaches the absorption site.

78	**a = A**	In *all* there are often no B- or T-cell markers, but some cases show immunoglobulin heavy-chain rearrangements indicating a B-cell origin.
	b = E	This enzyme histochemical reaction distinguishes monoblasts from myeloblasts.
	c = C	Leukaemic cells with cytoplasmic projections are found in hairy cell leukaemia, which is of B-cell origin (B).

Philadelphia chromosome (C) is a marker for chronic granulocytic leukaemia.

79   **E**   Chronic granulocytic leukaemia is the commonest cause of massive splenomegaly in the UK; splenomegaly does occur in the acute leukaemias but is seldom massive.

80	**a = D**	This rare condition involves a neoplastic proliferation of lymphoid cells in the mucosa of the small intestine; the cells produce alpha chain.
	b = A	Bence–Jones protein consists of light chains of immunoglobulin molecules; 15% of myelomas produce only light chains.
	c = B	Waldenstrom's macroglobulinaemia is a condition in which the neoplastic cells produce IgM which increases blood viscosity.

Increased red cell mass occurs in the myeloproliferative disorder polycythaemia rubra vera (C). A solitary tumour in a long bone is typical of a solitary plasmacytoma (E).

81   **E**   Secondary carcinoma is much more common than any of the others, which may all arise primarily in lymph nodes.

82 For each of the systemic diseases listed on the left select the most appropriate lymph node abnormality from the list on the right.
   a. Rheumatoid arthritis
   b. Psoriasis
   c. Toxoplasmosis

   A. Bizarre paracortical T-cell reaction
   B. Epithelioid granulomas in germinal centres
   C. Follicular hyperplasia with medullary plasma cells
   D. Lipid and melanin in paracortical histiocytes
   E. Palisaded necrotising granulomas

83 For each of the types of Hodgkin's disease listed on the left select the most appropriate histological feature from the list on the right.
   a. Lymphocyte predominance
   b. Mixed cellularity
   c. Nodular sclerosis

   A. Coarse bands of collagen
   B. Few Reed–Sternberg cells
   C. Fibrous tissue prominent
   D. Prominent eosinophils, plasma cells and macrophages
   E. Abundant Reed–Sternberg cells

84 If the following events were placed in chronological order which would come *fourth*?
   A. Biopsy of cervical lymph node
   B. Chemotherapy instituted
   C. Fungal infection of lungs
   D. Lymphadenopathy detected by GP
   E. Patient complains of night sweats

85 Which *one* of the following examples of non-Hodgkin's lymphoma commonly occurs in children?
   A. Diffuse centrocytic
   B. Follicular centroblastic/centrocytic
   C. Lymphoblastic lymphoma
   D. Lymphocytic lymphoma
   E. Lymphoplasmacytoid lymphoma

86 For each of the tumours listed on the left select the most appropriate association from the list on the right.
   a. Adenolymphoma
   b. Pleomorphic salivary adenoma
   c. Squamous carcinoma of oral mucosa

   A. Benign easily resectable tumour of the parotid gland
   B. High incidence of local recurrence
   C. Malignant tumour of parotid gland
   D. May arise in Sjogren's disease
   E. Prognosis depends on site

87 If the following events were placed in chronological order which would come *fourth*?
   A. Aspiration bronchopneumonia
   B. Difficulty in swallowing
   C. Heavy alcohol intake
   D. Oesophageal bouginage
   E. Tracheo-oesophageal fistula

82 **a = C** Hyperplasia of germinal centres with plasma cells in the paracortex is seen in patients with rheumatoid arthritis who develop enlargement of lymph nodes; splenomegaly may also occur.

    b = D Patients with skin diseases such as psoriasis or eczema may develop lymph node enlargement with melanin and lipid from the skin and dermis being filtered at the draining lymph node.

    c = B Infection with *Toxoplasma gondii* may result in enlarged lymph nodes in which there is sinus histiocytosis and granuloma formation. Bizarre paracortical T-cell reactions (A) may be seen in patients with glandular fever due to Epstein–Barr virus infection.
Necrotising granulomas with a peripheral palisade of histiocytes may be seen in cat-scratch disease (E). The causative organism is not known.

83 **a = B** In lymphocyte predominance Hodgkin's disease Reed–Sternberg cells are scanty, and the main cell type is the lymphocyte. This is the best prognostic type and may be a B-cell lymphoma.

    b = D Mixed cellularity Hodgkin's disease is characterised by Reed–Sternberg cells set in a mixed cell background.

    c = A In nodular sclerosis Hodgkin's disease, dense bands of collagen divide the node into nodules that contain lacunar cells.
Prominent fibrous tissue (C) and abundant Reed–Sternberg cells (E) are features of the poor-prognosis lymphocyte-depletion type.

84   **B** The patient complains of night sweats (E) to the GP who discovers enlarged lymph nodes (D) which are biopsied by the surgeon (A). The nodes are involved by Hodgkin's disease and the patient is treated by chemotherapy (B), which results in immunosuppression with opportunistic fungal infection supervening (C).

85   **C** The thymic or mediastinal lymphoblastic lymphoma of T-cell type affects males in late childhood or adolescence. The other types tend to occur in adults over 30 years.

86 **a = A** This occurs in middle-aged men and is often bilateral; it is benign. This is the second commonest parotid tumour.

    b = B Pleomorphic salivary adenomas are benign, but tend to extend through the capsule so that complete resection is not possible.

    c = E Intra-oral squamous carcinoma has a worsening prognosis the further back in the mouth it is.
Sjogren's disease (D) is an autoimmune disease, and a malignant lymphoma may arise in an affected salivary gland. Adenoid cystic carcinoma (C) is the commonest malignant salivary gland tumour.

87   **E** Heavy alcohol intake (C) is associated with the development of oesophageal carcinoma in Western Europe.
An early symptom of oesophageal carcinoma is dysphagia (B); surgical treatment may be impossible and palliative oesophageal bouginage undertaken (D). This may be complicated by oesophageal rupture, but occasionally the tumour itself extends locally into the trachea and a fistula is formed (E), with resultant aspiration bronchopneumonia (A).

88 For each of the forms of gastritis listed on the left select the most appropriate association from the list of histological features on the right.

   a. Acute gastritis
   b. Type A chronic gastritis
   c. Type B chronic gastritis

   A. Bacteria present in the superficial mucus layer
   B. Granulomatous inflammation of the mucosa
   C. Inflammation limited to the superficial mucosa
   D. Mucosa thin with intestinal metaplasia
   E. Mucosal hypertrophy

89 Which *one* of the following is *not* a predisposing factor for peptic ulcer?
   A. Achlorhydria
   B. Blood group O
   C. Cigarette smoking
   D. High gastrin secretion
   E. Ingestion of aspirin

90 For each of the features of gastric carcinoma listed on the left select the most appropriate association from the list on the right.

   a. Linitis plastica
   b. Signet ring cells
   c. Superficial spreading carcinoma

   A. Deep layers of stomach wall infiltrated and thickened
   B. Extensive spread in mucosa and submucosa
   C. Globule of mucin within tumour cell
   D. Nodular mass of tumour protruding into lumen
   E. Present in the edge of a gastric ulcer

91 For each of the pathological features noted on the left select the most appropriate disease from the list on the right.

   a. Colonic mucosal pseudopolyps
   b. Pericolic abscess in the left iliac fossa
   c. Small intestinal mucosa with cobblestone surface

   A. Appendicitis
   B. Crohn's disease
   C. Diverticulitis
   D. Diverticulosis
   E. Ulcerative colitis

92 For each of the organisms on the left select the most appropriate association from the list on the right.

   a. Campylobacter
   b. *Clostridium difficile*
   c. *Vibrio cholerae*

   A. Antibiotic-associated diarrhoea
   B. Enlargement of Peyer's patches
   C. Infective diarrhoea
   D. Stimulation of adenyl cyclase activity
   E. Stool examination often diagnostic

88 **a = C** Superficial epithelial erosion and limited inflammation are features of acute gastritis.

    b = D Type A (autoimmune gastritis) is associated with destruction of the specialised cells of the gastric glands and resultant atrophy and intestinal metaplasia.

    c = A *Helicobacter pylori* are the main feature of type B gastritis and are implicated in its pathogenesis.
Granulomatous (B) and hypertrophic (E) gastritis are rare.

89 **A** The presence of gastric acid is necessary for the development of peptic ulcer; in the stomach defective mucosal protection appears to be more important than the quantity of acid; in the duodenum gastric hypersecretion is more important.
There is a higher incidence of peptic ulcer in people of blood group O (B). Cigarette smoking (C) and ingestion of certain drugs (E) result in increased risk of ulcer. High gastrin secretion (D) from a pancreatic islet cell tumour results in a fulminating ulcer diathesis (Zollinger–Ellison syndrome).

90 **a = A** In this growth pattern the mucosa appears uninvolved grossly, the stomach wall becoming rigid due to tumour infiltration.

    b = C Signet ring cells are characteristic of gastric carcinoma but may be seen in other tumours also.

    c = B In this growth pattern there is no evidence of deep invasion, the tumour spreading widely in the superficial layers.
Gastric carcinoma has various growth patterns including nodular outgrowths (D) and large fungating ulcerated masses. Occasionally a carcinoma may arise in the edge of an ulcer (E); more commonly the ulcer is due to tumour necrosis.

91 **a = E** Pseudopolyps consist of surviving hyperplastic mucosa and granulation tissue.

    b = C Diverticulosis (D) is the presence of diverticulums, which are not inflamed; in diverticulitis they become inflamed and may rupture to produce pericolic abscesses. The symptoms are similar to those in appendicitis (A) but affect the left side.

    c = B The appearance of linear fissuring and ulceration of the oedematous mucosa of Crohn's disease gives the typical cobblestone pattern.

92 **a = C** Recently many cases of infective diarrhoea have been shown to be due to organisms of the Campylobacter group.

    b = A Antibiotic-associated diarrhoea (pseudomembranous colitis) is due to infection by *Clostridium difficile* and the effects of its toxin on the mucosa.

    c = D The vibrio toxin stimulates adenyl cyclase activity which alters fluid and electrolyte balance between mucosal cells and the gut lumen.
Enlargement of Peyer's patches is a feature of typhoid (B). Stool examination is essential for the diagnosis of amoebic dysentery (E).

93   Which *one* of the following is an example of a primary malabsorption syndrome?
     A. A-β-lipoproteinaemia
     B. Blind-loop syndrome
     C. Coeliac disease
     D. Crohn's disease
     E. Pancreatic insufficiency

94   Which *one* of the following conditions predisposes to colonic carcinoma?
     A. Bacillary dysentery
     B. Crohn's disease
     C. Diverticular disease
     D. Ischaemic colitis
     E. Ulcerative colitis

95   For each of the types of colonic polyp listed on the left select the most
     appropriate association from the list on the right.
     a. Tubular adenoma   A. Always shows invasion of the
     b. Tubulo-villous   stalk
        adenoma   B. Hamartomatous lesion
     c. Villous adenoma   C. High risk of undergoing
                                      malignant transformation
                                   D. Intermediate histological features
                                   E. Usually less than 10 mm in
                                      diameter

96   In which *one* of the following conditions is fatty change of the liver *not*
     a feature?
     A. Alcohol abuse
     B. Kwashiorkor
     C. Obesity
     D. Pernicious anaemia
     E. Viral hepatitis

97   Which *one* of the following is *not* usually a feature of acute viral hepatitis in a
     liver biopsy?
     A. Eosinophilic degeneration of hepatocytes
     B. Hepatocyte vacuolation
     C. Intact reticulin framework
     D. Lymphocytic infiltrate in parenchyma and portal tracts
     E. Mallory bodies

98   For each outcome of infection by hepatitis B (HB) virus on the left select the
     most appropriate association from the list on the right.
     a. Asymptomatic HB   A. Antimitochondrial antibody
        carrier with low   B. HBcAb and HBsAb produced
        infectivity   C. HBcAg and HBsAg both expressed
     b. HB positive chronic   by hepatocytes
        active hepatitis   D. Predominant HBcAg expression
     c. Recovery from acute   E. Predominant HBsAg expression in
        HB   serum and hepatocytes

93   **C**   Coeliac disease (gluten-sensitive enteropathy) is a primary malabsorption syndrome. The others are all causes of secondary malabsorption in that they interfere with absorption for various reasons: bacterial colonization in the blind-loop syndrome (B), severe mucosal damage in Crohn's disease (D).

Pancreatic insufficiency (E) causes inadequate digestion. A-β-lipoproteinaemia is a biochemical defect that interferes with absorption (A).

94   **E**   There is an increased risk of colonic carcinoma in patients with long-standing, extensive ulcerative colitis.

Crohn's disease (B) is associated with an increased risk of small intestinal malignancy, but this is rare.

95 **a = E**   Tubular adenomas are usually small rounded nodules on a stalk.

      b = D   Tubulo-villous adenomas show a mixed histological pattern and are intermediate in size between tubular and villous adenomas.

      c = C   Villous adenomas are usually sessile, larger than 10 mm in diameter and have a large surface area; these are most likely to become malignant.

Invasion of the stalk of a polyp is an important criterion of malignancy (A) but is not invariably present. If the stalk is twisted glandular tissue may be trapped in it giving rise to pseudoinvasion.

The juvenile polyp is a hamartomatous lesion of the mucosa (B).

96   **E**   Fatty change is not a feature in acute viral hepatitis.

All of the others involve nutritional deficiency and toxic damage to hepatocytes, which result in fatty change.

97   **E**   Mallory bodies are usually found in alcoholic hepatitis, but occur in other conditions, e.g. Indian childhood cirrhosis.

The others are the histological hallmarks of acute hepatitis; eosinophilic degeneration of hepatocytes (A) with extrusion of the pyknotic nucleus produces the Councilman body.

98 **a = E**   If virus is not completely eliminated a carrier state may develop with continued expression of HBsAg; this is viral envelope and is of low infectivity.

      b = C   In some cases chronic liver disease develops with continued expression of HBcAg and HBsAg.

      c = B   Successful elimination of virus with resolution of the hepatitis results from adequate humoral responses.

Antimitochondrial antibody (A) is present in primary biliary cirrhosis. Predominant HBcAg (D) expression occurs in carriers who remain highly infective.

99 For each of the features of alcoholic liver disease listed on the left select the
    most appropriate association from the list on the right.
    a. Fatty liver   A. Evidence of hepatocyte
    b. Alcoholic hepatitis   regeneration
    c. Micronodular   B. Ground glass hepatocytes
       cirrhosis   C. Hepatitis predominantly around
                                               hepatic vein branches
                                            D. Portal areas severely affected
                                               initially
                                            E. Recovery occurs if alcohol
                                               withdrawn

100 Oesophageal varices are caused by which *one* of the following?
    A. Enlarged liver pressing on the portal vein.
    B. Portal hypertension
    C. Pulmonary hypertension
    D. Systemic hypertension
    E. Tumour metastases in the porta hepatis

101 For each of the types of liver tumour listed on the left select the most
    appropriate association from the list on the right.
    a. Cholangiocarcinoma   A. Commonest primary liver tumour
    b. Haemangiosarcoma   B. Exposure to vinyl chloride
    c. Liver cell adenoma   monomer
                                            C. Sex hormone therapy
                                            D. Tumour of childhood
                                            E. Ulcerative colitis

102 With which *one* of the following do gallstones and/or chronic cholecystitis *not*
    have a recognized association?
    A. Acute pancreatitis
    B. Haemolytic anaemia
    C. Hepatitis B infection
    D. Intestinal obstruction
    E. Typhoid fever

103 For each of the pancreatic lesions listed on the left select the most appropiate
    association from the list on the right.
    a. Acute pancreatitis   A. Autosomal dominant inheritance
    b. Chronic pancreatitis   B. Exocrine pancreas atrophy
    c. Pancreatic   C. Migrating thrombophlebitis
       adenocarcinoma   D. Raised serum amylase
                                            E. Recurrent peptic ulceration

104 If the following events were placed in chronological order which would come
    fourth?
    A. Cingulate gyrus herniates beneath falx cerebri
    B. Frontal lobe tumour in right hemisphere
    C. Interventricular septum shifts to left of midline
    D. Medial temporal lobe herniates through tentorial opening
    E. Pontine and midbrain haemorrhage

99   **a = E**   The metabolic effects of alcohol on hepatocytes responsible for fatty change are reversible if alcohol is stopped. This is the earliest feature of alcoholic liver damage.

     b = C   The site of earliest damage in alcoholic liver disease is around the terminal hepatic vein (centrilobular); hepatocyte necrosis in this area is very suggestive of alcohol damage.

     c = A   Before cirrhosis can be present hepatocyte regeneration has to occur, along with fibrosis; fibrosis on its own is not cirrhosis. Ground glass hepatocytes (B) are a feature of hepatitis B infection. The portal areas (D) are affected later in alcoholic hepatitis when extensive damage has occurred and when cirrhosis is present.

100   **B**   Portal hypertension (mainly caused by cirrhosis) results from interference with the hepatic micro-circulation such that vessels in the portal-systemic anastomotic system become engorged and develop varicosities. This occurs most spectacularly in the oesophagus and rupture of these veins is a common cause of death in alcoholics.

101   **a = E**   Patients with ulcerative colitis may develop sclerosing cholangitis, which is associated with the development of cholangiocarcinoma. In the Far East infection by liver fluke causes this tumour.

     b = B   Exposure to vinyl chloride monomer is implicated in the development of this tumour.

     c = C   Oral contraceptive and sex hormone therapy has been associated with the development of these benign liver cell tumours. The commonest primary liver cell tumour (A) is the hepatocellular carcinoma. The hepatoblastoma is a liver cell tumour of childhood (D).

102   **C**   There is no association with viral hepatitis. Haemolytic anaemia (B) is associated with the formation of pigment stones. The presence of gallstones is associated with pancreatitis and rarely with small intestinal obstruction (D). Typhoid fever may result in a carrier state in which organisms survive in the gallbladder (E).

103   **a = D**   This is a diagnostic test for acute pancreatitis; the release of amylase is also responsible for the clinicopathological features of pancreatitis.

     b = B   In this condition there is fibrosis of the pancreas with atrophy of the exocrine pancreas.

     c = C   Migrating thrombophlebitis is one of the bizarre clinical effects seen in patients with pancreatic cancer. Recurrent peptic ulceration (E) is a feature of the endocrine pancreatic tumours that secrete gastrin.

104   **D**   A tumour in the right frontal lobe (B) will act as a space-occupying lesion resulting in raised intracranial pressure; expansion of the right hemisphere causes shift of the midline (C), the cingulate gyrus herniates beneath the falx (A); increasing expansion results in a tentorial hernia (D) and eventually fatal pontine and midbrain haemorrhage (E) supervene.

105 For each of the types of haematoma listed on the left select the most
appropriate association from the list on the right.
   a. Acute subdural haematoma   A. Associated with cerebral
   b. Chronic subdural haematoma   contusions and lacerations in
   c. Extradural haematoma   many cases
                                      B. Due to rupture of an aneurysm.
                                      C. May present weeks after trivial
                                         injury
                                      D. Scarring of frontal poles
                                      E. Usually due to a tear of the
                                         middle meningeal artery

106 Which *one* of the following is *not* a common site of hypertensive intracerebral
haemorrhage?
   A. Basal ganglia
   B. Cerebellum
   C. Internal capsule
   D. Occipital poles
   E. Pons

107 Which *one* of the following is *not* a common site of a saccular (berry) aneurysm?
   A. Basilar artery
   B. Bifurcation of the middle cerebral artery
   C. Junction of anterior communicating artery and anterior cerebral artery
   D. Junction of internal carotid artery and posterior communicating artery
   E. Vertebral artery

108 If the following events were placed in chronological order which would come
fourth?
   A. Abscess in temporal lobe
   B. Chronic otitis media
   C. Inadequate antibiotic therapy
   D. Invasion of venous channels by bacteria
   E. Osteitis of the tegmen tympani

109 For each of the types of virus infection listed on the left select the most
appropriate association from the list on the right.
   a. Cytomegalovirus.   A. Anterior horn motor cells
   b. Herpes simplex virus.   B. Bilateral temporal lobe
   c. Type 1   necrosis
      poliomyelitis virus.   C. Inclusion body in Purkinje cell
                                       cytoplasm
                                   D. Nuclear inclusion bodies found
                                       in periventricular cells
                                   E. Spongiform encephalopathy

110 For each of the conditions listed on the left select the most appropriate
association from the list on the right.
   a. Acute disseminated   A. Complication of septic shock
      perivenous   B. Complication of smallpox
      encephalomyelitis   vaccination
   b. Acute haemorrhagic   C. Experimental model for
      leucoencephalitis   demyelinating diseases
   c. Multiple sclerosis   D. Familial disease due to enzyme
                                       deficiency
                                    E. Unilateral optic neuritis is an
                                       early symptom

105 **a = A**   This is a common finding if death occurs soon after a head injury which causes severe damage to cerebral tissue.

   b = C   Trivial injury (particularly in the elderly) may result in slow haemorrhage from the bridging veins, which produces a slowly expanding haematoma.

   c = E   Fracture of the skull, particularly the temporal bone, may result in tearing of a meningeal vessel; classically there is a lucid interval followed by headache, drowsiness and coma.
   Rupture of a an aneurysm (B) usually produces a subarachnoid haemorrhage. Scarring (D) is a sign of previous head injury.

106   **D**   Hypertensive intracerebral haemorrhage usually results from a rupture of a microaneurysm on a perforating cerebral artery; the commonest sites are basal ganglia (A), internal capsule (C), pons (E) and cerebellum (B).

107   **E**   Saccular (berry, or congenital) aneurysms are due to a defect in the medial coat at sites of bifurcation of the intracerebral arteries; the commonest sites are middle cerebral bifurcation (B), anterior communicator and anterior cerebral (C), internal carotid and posterior communicator (D) and on the basilar artery (A). These aneurysms are often multiple.

108   **D**   Chronic otitis media (B) inadequately treated (C) may result in inflammation of the surrounding bone (E); this allows invasion of the venous channels by bacteria (D), which gain access to the brain producing an abscess (A).

109 **a = D**   Cytomegalovirus infection of the CNS is usually acquired *in utero* and is characterised by intranuclear inclusion bodies.

   b = B   Herpes simplex infection of the CNS gives asymmetrical temporal lobe necrosis (acute necrotising encephalitis).

   c = A   Poliomyelitis affects the motor cells of the anterior horns of the spinal cord.
   Inclusion bodies in the cytoplasm of the Purkinje cells of the cerebellum (C) are a diagnostic feature of rabies (Negri bodies). Spongiform encephalopathy is found in slow virus infections (Kuru and Creutzfeldt–Jacob disease) and may be caused by prions.

110 **a = B**   This condition follows viral infections such as measles, rubella and may complicate smallpox vaccination.

   b = A   This condition may follow virus infection or may complicate septic shock.

   c = E   An early symptom in the relapsing course of multiple sclerosis may be optic neuritis.
   Experimental auto-allergic encephalomyelitis (EAE) is a model for demyelinating diseases (C). There are several familial diseases due to enzyme deficiencies which cause abnormalities of myelination (D); metachromatic leukodystrophy is a deficiency of arylsulphatase A.

111 For each of the conditions listed on the left select the most appropriate
    association from the list on the right.
    a. Amyotrophic lateral   A. Damage to lower motor neurones
       sclerosis   in spinal cord
    b. Progressive bulbar   B. Damage to lower motor neurones
       palsy   in medulla
    c. Progressive muscular   C. Damage to posterior and lateral
       atrophy   columns
                                    D. Impaired blood flow in anterior
                                       spinal artery
                                    E. Upper and lower motor neurone
                                       damage

112 Which *one* of the following is the commonest intracerebral neoplasm?
    A. Astrocytoma
    B. Ependymoma
    C. Meningioma
    D. Oligodendroglioma
    E. Secondary carcinoma

113 Which *one* of the following forms a cystic tumour mass in the cerebellum in
    children?
    A. Astrocytoma
    B. Ependymoma
    C. Glioblastoma multiforme
    D. Haemangioblastoma
    E. Medulloblastoma

114 Which *one* of the following is characteristically found in acute diffuse
    proliferative glomerulonephritis?
    A. Endothelial and mesangial cell hyperplasia
    B. Fibrinoid necrosis of glomerular capillaries
    C. Focal sclerosis of glomerular tufts
    D. Hyalinisation of arcuate arteries
    E. Severe basement membrane thickening

115 Rapidly progressive glomerulonephritis is best characterized morphologically by
    which *one* of the following?
    A. Basement membrane thickening
    B. Crescent formation
    C. Fibrinoid necrosis of the afferent arteriole
    D. Interstitial fibrosis
    E. Mesangial cell proliferation

116 For each of the ultrastructural features of glomerulonephritis listed on the left
    select the most appropriate association from the list on the right.
    a. Dense deposits in   A. Acute diffuse glomerulonephritis
       outer part of the   B. Focal glomerulonephritis
       basement membrane   C. Membranous glomerulonephritis
    b. Dense subepithelial   D. Mesangiocapillary
       deposits   glomerulonephritis
    c. Fusion of   E. Minimal change
       epithelial cell   glomerulonephritis
       foot processes

111 **a = E**   This variant of motor neurone disease involves degeneration of both upper and lower motor neurones.

b = B   In bulbar palsy the lower motor neurones of the medulla are affected.

c = A   In progressive muscular atrophy the spinal cord and lower motor neurones are affected.

Damage to posterior and lateral tracts is a feature of Friedrich's ataxia (C). Acute myelitis may be caused by vascular insufficiency in the spinal cord (D).

112   **E**   The commonest intracerebral neoplasms are secondaries.
Astrocytoma (A) is the commonest type of glioma.
Ependymoma (B) is found in children; meningioma (C) originates from the arachnoid granulations and presses into the brain tissue from outside.

113   **A**   Cerebellar astrocytomas in children are usually cystic.
Glioblastoma multiforme (C) is an anaplastic astrocytoma, which occurs in the cerebral hemisphere of adults. Medulloblastoma (E) is derived from nerve cells and occurs in the cerebellum of children; it is not usually cystic.
Haemangioblastoma (D) is a tumour of blood vessels and occurs usually in the cerebellum.

114   **A**   The characteristic finding in this type of glomerulonephritis is enlargement and hypercellularity of the glomeruli, contributed to by capillary endothelial cell and mesangial cell hyperplasia.
Fibrinoid necrosis of glomerular capillaries (B) and hyalinisation of arcuate arteries (D) are seen in malignant phase hypertension. Focal sclerosis (C) of glomerular tufts is seen in focal glomerulosclerosis.
Basement membrane thickening (E) is seen in membranous glomerulonephritis.

115   **B**   Proliferation of the parietal epithelium of Bowman's capsule forms epithelial crescents which obliterate the capsular space; the crescents also contain macrophages.
Interstitial fibrosis can have many causes but is seen where there is loss of glomeruli with resultant atrophy of the nephron (D).

116 **a = C**   The dense deposits on the basement membrane are the 'spikes' seen on the basement membrane by light microscopy; they consist of IgG and complement.

b = A   The subepithelial deposits consist of IgG and complement and represent trapped small immune complexes.

c = E   The only feature of note in minimal change disease is fusion of the epithelial cell foot processes.
In mesangiocapillary glomerulonephritis (D) there are two types of ultrastructural change – type 1 consists of subendothelial deposits; type 2 is dense deposit disease.

117 Which *one* of the following is *not* a feature of diabetic kidneys?
   A. Crystals in the collecting tubules
   B. Hyaline nodules at the periphery of the glomerular tuft
   C. Hyaline thickening of the glomerular capillary basement membrane
   D. Ischaemic glomerular collapse
   E. Papillary necrosis

118 For each of the features listed on the left select the most appropriate cause from the list on the right.
   a. Irregular cortical
      scars related to a
      deformed calyx
   b. Multiple small
      abscesses in renal cortex
   c. Streaks of
      suppuration extending
      from the papillae

   A. Acute pyelonephritis
   B. Chronic pyelonephritis
   C. Infective endocarditis
   D. Renal artery stenosis
   E. Systemic hypertension

119 Which *one* of the following is *not* a feature of clear cell carcinoma of the kidney?
   A. Bony secondaries
   B. Childhood tumour
   C. Haematuria
   D. May appear encapsulated
   E. Renal vein invasion

120 For each of the conditions listed on the left select the most appropriate association from the list on the right.
   a. Bilateral
      hydronephrosis
   b. Pyonephrosis
   c. Unilateral
      hydronephrosis

   A. Aberrant renal vein
   B. Infected staghorn calculus
   C. Michaelis-Gutmann bodies
   D. Narrowing at pelvi-ureteric
      junction
   E. Urethral obstruction

121 Which *one* of the following is the commonest type of bladder tumour?
   A. Adenocarcinoma
   B. Lymphoma
   C. Papillary transitional cell carcinoma
   D. Solid transitional cell carcinoma
   E. Squamous carcinoma

122 For each of the conditions listed on the left select the most appropriate association from the list on the right.
   a. Osteomalacia
   b. Renal osteodystrophy
   c. Rickets

   A. Failure of mineralization of
      cartilage of epiphyseal growth
      plate
   B. Nephrocalcinosis
   C. Osteoid borders around calcified
      trabeculae
   D. Osteitis fibrosa with
      osteomalacia and osteoclerosis
   E. Subperiosteal new bone formation
      in several bones

117   **A**   Crystals in the collecting tubules are a feature of gout. Hyaline nodules (Kimmelstiel–Wilson) are seen in nodular glomerulosclerosis (B). Basement membrane thickening (C) is seen in diffuse glomerulosclerosis.

As a result of hyaline thickening of the afferent arterioles ischaemic glomerular damage may occur (D).

Papillary necrosis (E) is commonly seen in diabetic kidneys.

118 **a = B**   The relationship between cortical scars and calyceal scars is important in differentiating the scarred kidneys of pyelonephritis from other causes of scarring, e.g. hypertension (E).

    b = C   Infective endocarditis results in septic emboli which cause pyaemic abscesses in the kidneys.

    c = A   Acute inflammation of the pelvis associated with streaks of pus extending along the medullary rays to the cortex is seen in acute pyelonephritis.

Renal artery stenosis (D) results in a uniform contraction of the kidney, usually unilateral.

119   **B**   The nephroblastoma is a childhood renal tumour. Clear cell carcinomas may appear encapsulated (D) but are malignant and often show renal vein invasion (E) with resultant lung and bone secondaries (A). Haematuria occurs if they extend into the pelvis (C).

120 **a = E**
    b = B   Infection of the renal pelvis is often associated with the presence of a calculus in the pelvis.

    c = D   Other causes of unilateral hydronephrosis include impaction of a stone in the ureter, the presence of a ureteric tumour or an aberrant renal artery (not vein, A).

Michaelis-Gutmann bodies (C) are seen in malacoplakia.

121   **C**   Papillary transitional cell carcinoma is the commonest bladder neoplasm. Solid variants (D) occur and are usually of a higher grade, and worse prognosis.

Squamous carcinoma (E) may arise from squamous metaplasia of transitional epithelium or directly from transitional epithelium. Adenocarcinoma (A) and lymphoma (B) are rare.

122 **a = C**   Vitamin D deficiency results in failure of calcium absorption and hence failure of calcification of osteoid matrix, which is laid down around already mineralised bone.

    b = D   Renal osteodystrophy shows a complex pattern of bony changes secondary to chronic renal failure.

    c = A   Rickets is the childhood equivalent of osteomalacia; there is failure of mineralization of the cartilage of the epiphyseal growth plate and this results in deformity.

Nephrocalcinosis (B) occurs in infantile hypercalcaemia. Subperiosteal new bone formation at several sites (E) is the hallmark of the 'battered baby' syndrome.

123 For each of the conditions listed on the left select the most appropriate association from the list on the right.

a. Osteoporosis
b. Paget's disease of bone
c. Primary hyperparathyroidism

A. Collections of eosinophils
B. Decrease in amount of bone with normal mineralisation of matrix
C. Fibrous tissue around and within trabeculae
D. High proportion of woven to lamellar bone
E. Mosaic pattern of cement lines

124 If the following were placed in chronological order which would come *fourth*?
A. Formation of involucrum
B. Localised skin infection
C. Sequestrum formation
D. Subperiosteal abscess
E. Suppuration of medullary cavity

125 Which *one* of the following is the commonest tumour in bone?
A. Benign chondroblastoma
B. Chondrosarcoma
C. Giant cell tumour
D. Secondary carcinoma
E. Osteosarcoma

126 Which *one* of the following is *not* a feature of osteosarcoma?
A. 50% occur around the knee
B. Lung secondaries are common
C. May be associated with Paget's disease of bone
D. Peak incidence between 10 and 25 years of age
E. Usually metastasize to lymph nodes

127 For each of the types of tumour listed on the left select the most appropriate association from the list on the right.

a. Chondrosarcoma
b. Chordoma
c. Ewing's tumour

A. Giant cells are a prominent feature
B. Large cystic tumour arising in buttock
C. Sacrococcygeal tumour consisting of large pale cells
D. Tumour cells may contain glycogen
E. Urinary catecholamines elevated

128 Which *one* of the following is *not* a feature of rheumatoid arthritis?
A. Foreign body giant cell reaction to crystals
B. Frondose, inflamed synovium
C. Necrosis of subcutaneous collagen
D. Pannus formation
E. Prominent lymphoid follicle formation within hypertrophied synovial villi

123 **a = B** This may be due to decreased bone formation, increased resorption or a combination.

 b = E The mosaic pattern indicates a disturbance of normal resorption and reconstruction.

 c = C Osteitis fibrosa is a feature of hyperparathyroidism in which there is osteoclastic resorption of the centres of trabeculae with fibrous replacement and surrounding fibrosis.
Collections of eosinophils in bone (A) are seen in eosinophil granuloma.
Bone is poorly formed in the hereditary condition osteogenesis imperfecta (D) due to a mutation in the structural gene for type 1 collagen.

124 **C** A minor skin infection often caused by penicillin resistant *Staphylococcus aureus* (B) results in blood spread to the bone marrow (E) from where infection spreads through the cortical bone to produce a subperiosteal abscess (D); the presence of pus may result in thrombosis of the nutrient artery which causes death of the diaphyseal bone which forms the sequestrum (C). New bone is produced under the periosteum, forming an encasing sheath of irregular outline, the involucrum (A).

125 **D** Secondary tumours are more common than primary bone tumours, occurring in 70% of patients with disseminated malignant disease.

126 **E** Lymph node metastases are a feature of carcinoma rather than sarcoma, and osteosarcomas usually metastasize to the lung (B). The usual site for osteosarcoma is in a long bone, the femur and tibia being especially common (A). Osteosarcoma is a tumour of young people (D) but may occur in the elderly when it is usually associated with Paget's disease of bone (C).

127 **a = B** Chondrosarcomas are often bulky, gelatinous cystic tumours arising from the pelvic bones.

 b = C Chordomas arise in the sacrococcygeal region or at the spheno-occipital region; the tumour cells often contain droplets of mucoid material.

 c = D Ewing's tumour usually occurs in children and consists of sheets of small cells, which may contain glycogen. Giant cells are a feature of the giant cell tumour of bone or osteoclastoma (A). Urinary catecholamines are elevated (E) in neuroblastoma, a childhood tumour which may be difficult to distinguish from Ewing's tumour histologically.

128 **A** A foreign body giant cell reaction to crystals is characteristic of gout.

129 Osteoarthritis most commonly affects which *one* of the following sites?
   A. Ankle joint
   B. Costochondral joint
   C. Knee joint
   D. Metacarpophalangeal joint
   E. Proximal interphalangeal joint

130 For each of the conditions listed on the left select the most appropriate association from the list on the right.
   a. Malignant fibrous histiocytoma
   b. Myositis ossificans
   c. Rhabdomyosarcoma

   A. Commonest benign tumour of soft tissues
   B. Commonest sarcoma of late adult life
   C. Commonest soft tissue sarcoma of children
   D. Follows muscular injury
   E. Results in deformity of hand

131 If the following clinical and pathological features were in chronological order which would come *fourth*?
   A. Cervical biopsy shows cervical intraepithelial neoplasia, grade III
   B. Cone biopsy of cervix shows invasive squamous carcinoma
   C. Early onset of sexual activity
   D. Frozen pelvis
   E. Ureteric obstruction with uraemia

132 For each of the conditions listed on the left select the most appropriate association from those listed on the right.
   a. Atypical hyperplasia of the endometrium
   b. Endometrial adenocarcinoma
   c. Mixed homologous sarcoma

   A. Aberrant endometrial tissue
   B. Confined to uterus until a late stage
   C. Irregular glandular proliferation without stromal proliferation
   D. Proliferation of glandular and stromal endometrium
   E. Tumour of endometrial stromal and glandular origin

133 For each of the types of ovarian tumour listed on the left select the most appropriate association from the list on the right.
   a. Cystic teratoma
   b. Granulosa cell tumour
   c. Mucinous cystadenoma

   A. Associated with virilisation
   B. Benign tumour of germ cell origin
   C. Histologically identical to seminoma
   D. May cause endometrial hyperplasia
   E. Pseudomyxoma peritonei

129   **C**   Osteoarthritis affects principally large load bearing joints, the knee and hip being most severely affected. Smaller joints develop osteoarthritis as a result of repeated trauma.
The small joints of the hand (D, E) are the usual site of rheumatoid arthritis.

130   **a = B**   This tumour recurs after surgery, and has a high incidence of metastases.
    b = D   This is a benign condition that histologically may be confused with osteosarcoma.
    c = C   This is derived from striated muscle, and the cells are identified by the presence of cross striations or by electron microscopy.
The commonest benign tumour of soft tissues is a lipoma (A).
Dupuytren's contracture results in deformity of the hand (E).

131   **D**   Early onset of sexual activity and promiscuous sexual activity (C) are associated with increased risk of cervical cancer; biopsy of the cervix (A) shows CIN III. An excision or cone biopsy of the cervix is performed (B) that reveals invasive carcinoma; cervical carcinoma invades locally in the pelvis (D) and eventually causes uraemia by ureteric obstruction (E). Human papilloma virus types 16 and 18 have been implicated in the aetiology of cervical cancer.

132   **a = C**   This is associated with increased risk of progression to endometrial carcinoma.
    b = B   Due to the thickness of the myometrium invasive endometrial carcinoma remains confined to the uterus for a long time.
    c = E   Stromal sarcomas may be pure or mixed (i.e. contain adenocarcinoma). Homologous tumours contain only stromal cells; heterologous tumours contain extrauterine components.
Aberrant endometrial tissue (A) present in ovaries, fallopian tubes, appendix, etc. is known as endometriosis. Proliferation of glandular and stromal endometrial tissue (D) occurs in cystic glandular hyperplasia, which is not a premalignant condition.

133   **a = B**   Ovarian cystic teratomas are invariably benign and contain a mixture of well-differentiated tissues.
This is the commonest ovarian tumour (15–20%).
    b = D   The granulosa cell tumour is derived from the sex cord stroma and frequently secretes oestrogen, producing precocious puberty, endometrial hyperplasia and cancer.
    c = E   Mucinous cystadenomas are benign, but may rupture shedding seedlings of mucin-secreting neoplastic cells into the peritoneal cavity.
Virilisation (A) occurs with sex cord tumours which secrete androgens (androblastomas or Sertoli–Leydig cell tumours.
The dysgerminoma is identical to the seminoma (C).

134 For each of the conditions listed on the left select the most appropriate
    association from the list on the right.
    a. Choriocarcinoma   A. Atypical trophoblastic
    b. Ectopic pregnancy   proliferation
    c. Hydatidiform mole   B. Chromosomal constitution YY
                                      C. Common tumour in Great Britain
                                      D. May occur with an intrauterine
                                         contraceptive device *in situ*
                                      E. Neoplastic allograft in mother

135 Which *one* of the following is *not* a feature of fibrocystic change of the breast?
    A. Apocrine metaplasia of glandular epithelium
    B. Cyst formation
    C. Formation of new breast lobules
    D. Paget's disease of nipple
    E. Sclerosing adenosis

136 For each of the types of breast tumour listed on the left select the most
    appropriate association from the list on the right.
    a. Ductal carcinoma-   A. Bleeding from nipple
       in-situ   B. Heavy lymphocyte infiltrate
    b. Giant fibroadenoma   C. May progress to sarcoma
    c. Medullary carcinoma   D. Multiple small nodules
                                      E. Pre-invasive neoplasm

137 Which *one* of the following is *not* true of prostatic carcinoma?
    A. Acid phosphatase level raised in serum
    B. Alkaline phosphatase detected in tumour cells
    C. Metastases are osteoplastic
    D. Microacinar carcinoma
    E. Usually arises in periphery of gland

138 Which *one* of the following is *not* true of benign nodular hyperplasia of the
    prostate gland?
    A. Commences around the urethra
    B. Effects are due to stenosis of the urethra
    C. Hyperplasia involves epithelium and stroma
    D. Incidence increases with age
    E. Under hormonal influence

139 For each of the types of testicular tumour listed on the left select the most
    appropriate association from the list on the right.
    a. Differentiated   A. Commonest testicular tumour in
       teratoma   the elderly
    b. Malignant teratoma   B. Consists of sheets of large pale
       intermediate   cells and lymphocytes
    c. Seminoma   C. Consists of trophoblastic
                                         elements
                                      D. Consists of a mixture of
                                         undifferentiated
                                         and differentiated tissues.
                                      E. Very rare tumour

134 **a = E**   This is a malignant tumour of cyto- and syncytiotrophoblast and is of purely fetal origin.

   b = D   Ectopic pregnancy usually results from a tubal abnormality but the risk is increased in women who become pregnant with an IUCD *in situ.*

   c = A   In hydatidiform mole there is abnormal development of trophoblast which is genetically of paternal origin and has chromosomal pattern XX.
   Choriocarcinoma is a rare tumour in Great Britain (C) but is common in the Far East.

135   **D**   Paget's disease of the nipple is intraepithelial spread of breast cancer. It occurs when ductal carcinoma spreads along major ducts to the nipple.

136 **a = E**   In DCIS the malignant cells are confined within the ducts.

   b = C   Giant fibroadenoma occurs in older women and may undergo malignant transformation to a sarcoma.

   c = B   This variant of breast cancer is characterized by sheets of malignant cells with a lymphocytic infiltrate that may be responsible for a slightly better prognosis.
   Bleeding from the nipple (A) is seen in papillomas of the nipple ducts. Benign fibroadenomas often present as multiple small nodules (D) in the breast.

137   **B**   Alkaline phosphatase is not produced by prostatic carcinoma, although the presence of bone metastases (C) may result in a rise in serum alkaline phosphatase. Acid phosphatase (A) of prostatic origin can be detected in the serum in many cases, as can prostate specific antigen.

138   **B**   The prostatic urethra is distorted by BNH, but the urinary symptoms are due to disturbance of the bladder sphincter mechanism rather than organic stenosis.

139 **a = E**   This type of tumour resembles the ovarian cystic teratoma, but is malignant; it is the rarest type of teratoma.

   b = D   This type involves a complex mixture of differentiated tissues, often with an 'organoid' structure, and undifferentiated tumour.

   c = B   This is the commonest type of testicular tumour, occurring usually in the fourth and fifth decades.
   The commonest testicular tumour in the elderly (A) is a lymphoma. A teratoma consisting of trophoblastic elements (C) resembles choriocarcinoma and may secrete HCG, which is used as a serum marker.

140 For each effect on the left select the most appropriate pituitary lesion from the
list on the right.
   a. Acromegaly   A. Craniopharyngioma
   b. Cushing's syndrome   B. GH-immunoreactive adenoma
   c. Sheehan's syndrome   C. Hyaline change in non-tumourous
                                            pituicytes
                                         D. Post-partum necrosis
                                         E. Rathke's cyst

141 For each of the thyroid conditions on the left select the most appropriate
association from the list on the right.
   a. Hyperthyroidism   A. Adenoma
   b. Hypothyroidism   B. Autoimmune disease
   c. Non-toxic nodular   C. Dyshormonogenesis
      goitre   D. Graves' disease
                                         E. Iodine deficiency

142 For each feature on the left select the most appropriate association from the list
on the right.
   a. Multiple peptic   A. Adrenocortical adenoma
      ulcers   B. Islet cell tumour of pancreas
   b. Nephrocalcinosis   C. Phaeochromocytoma
   c. Virilisation   D. Parathyroid adenoma
                                         E. Thyroid adenoma

143 Which *one* of the following is *most* likely to lead to blood borne metastases?
   A. Follicular carcinoma of thyroid
   B. Giant cell carcinoma of thyroid
   C. Medullary carcinoma of thyroid
   D. Papillary carcinoma of thyroid
   E. Small cell anaplastic carcinoma of thyroid

144 Which *one* of the following is *not* a virus infection of the skin?
   A. Condyloma acuminatum
   B. Molluscum contagiosum
   C. Pemphigus vulgaris
   D. Verruca vulgaris
   E. Zoster

145 Dermatitis herpetiformis is associated with which *one* of the following
conditions?
   A. Ankylosing spondylitis
   B. Diverticulitis
   C. Emphysema
   D. Gluten sensitive enteropathy
   E. Whipple's disease

140 **a = B**   Adenomas that secrete growth hormone produce acromegaly in adults, and gigantism when present before the epiphyses fuse.

      b = C   Excess ACTH results in increased production of glucocorticoids by the adrenals. Hyaline change is found in the corticotrophs - it is due to cytokeratin intermediate filaments.

      c = D   Post-partum hypotension results in ischaemic necrosis of the enlarged pituitary of pregnancy; this results in panhypopituitarism.
Craniopharingioma (C) and Rathke's cyst (E) are benign lesions of the suprasellar region, which may result in anterior pituitary damage by pressure necrosis.

141 **a = D**   Graves' disease is caused by excessive secretion of T3 and T4, as a result of diffuse thyroid hyperplasia caused by thyroid stimulating immunoglobulin.

      b = B   Autoimmune thyroiditis is characterized by lymphoid infiltration and destruction of thyroid acini; Hashimoto's disease is the commonest type.

      c = E   Iodine deficiency is the commonest cause of non-toxic goitre.
Dyshormonogenesis (C) results from genetically programmed lack of an essential enzyme, e.g. dehalogenase. Approximately 1% of adenomas (A) are functional.

142 **a = B**   Islet cell tumours of the pancreas may secrete gastrin which results in hypersecretion of gastric acid with resultant gastric and intestinal peptic ulceration (Zollinger–Ellison syndrome).

      b = D   Primary hyperparathyroidism is a result of parathyroid adenoma, which results in hypercalcaemia, and deposition of calcium in and around renal tubules.

      c = A   An adrenocortical adenoma may result in abnormal development due to excess secretion of androgens. Virilisation may also occur due to an enzyme deficiency (21-hydroxylase).
Phaeochromocytomas produce hypertension (C).

143   **A**   Follicular carcinoma has a propensity for invasion of capsular small blood vessels and early blood borne spread.

144   **C**   Pemphigus vulgaris is an inflammatory condition characterized by the presence of intra-epidermal bullous formation; there is circulating IgG class antibody to intercellular substance of squamous carcinoma.

145   **D**   The majority of patients with dermatitis herpetiformis have small intestinal villus abnormalities that respond to gluten withdrawal.

146 For each of the types of skin lesion listed on the left select the most appropriate association from the list on the right.
    a. Basal cell carcinoma
    b. Bowen's disease
    c. Solar keratosis

    A. Squamous carcinoma-in-situ on the legs
    B. Squamous carcinoma-in-situ on sun-exposed skin
    C. Tumour of sweat gland
    D. Tumour-like self-healing lesion
    E. Very rarely metastasizes

147 For each of the types of pigmented skin lesions listed on the left select the most appropriate association from the list on the right.
    a. Compound pigmented naevus
    b. Lentigo maligna
    c. Nodular melanoma

    A. Growth phase vertical only
    B. Increase in basal layer melanocytes
    C. Melanocytes in dermis and epidermis
    D. Presents on soles of feet.
    E. Slow-growing flat pigmented lesion

148 For each of the features of malaria listed on the left select the most appropriate association from the list on the right.
    a. Blackwater fever
    b. Malignant tertian fever
    c. Tropical splenomegaly syndrome

    A. Acute intravascular haemolysis
    B. Overwhelming parasitaemia with shock
    C. Pericapillary ring haemorrhages
    D. Regresses with long-term anti-malarial therapy
    E. Release of merozoites from burst RBC

149 For each of the lesions listed on the left select the most appropriate association from the list on the right.
    a. Leishman–Donovan bodies in Kupffer cells
    b. Meningo-encephalitis
    c. Self-healing ulcer

    A. African trypanosomiasis
    B. Cutaneous leishmaniasis
    C. Mucocutaneous leishmaniasis
    D. South American trypanosomiasis
    E. Visceral leishmaniasis

150 If the following events were placed in chronological order which would come *fourth*?
    A. Hepatic abscess formation
    B. Ingestion of contaminated water
    C. Lysis of epithelial cells in caecum
    D. Release of motile trophozoites
    E. Trophozoites enter portal blood

146 a = E Basal cell carcinomas (rodent ulcers) are locally aggressive and destructive tumours which very rarely metastasize.

b = A Carcinoma-in-situ of the skin may develop in areas not exposed to sun; it rarely becomes invasive carcinoma.

c = B Solar damage to the skin results in dysplasia, which may progress to invasive carcinoma in 20% of cases.

147 a = C Pigmented naevi are benign conditions in which there are increased numbers of melanocytes; the compound naevus is the commonest type in childhood.

b = E The lentigo maligna is essentially a malignant melanoma-in-situ.

c = A Malignant melanoma have a horizontal and vertical growth phase; nodular melanoma appears to have a vertical phase with no preceding horizontal phase.

Increased basal layer melanocytes are seen in a lentigo (B). A malignant melanoma which presents on the soles or palms is known as an acral lentiginous melanoma (D).

148 a = A Acute haemolysis occurs in non-immune patients following quinine treatment for falciparum malaria.

b = E Fever in malaria is either tertian (every 2 days) or quartan (every 3 days) and is due to release of merozoites from RBCs. Malignant tertian fever is due to *Plasmodium falciparum*.

c = D Splenomegaly may occur in adults with falciparum malaria; its pathogenesis is uncertain (hyper-reactive malarial splenomegaly).

Overwhelming parasitaemia with vascular collapse (B) is seen in algid malaria shock syndrome. Pericapillary ring haemorrhages are seen in cerebral malaria (C).

149 a = E In visceral leishmaniasis ('kala-azar') the organisms infect macrophages.

b = A In African trypanosomiasis the flagellates stay in the circulation, enter the central nervous system and alter the sleep rhythm.

c = B In cutaneous leishmaniasis a papule develops at the site of the insect bite and ulcerates, forming a crater.

In mucocutaneous leishmaniasis (C) non-healing secondary ulcers occur months or years after the primary lesion. South American trypanosomiasis (D) is characterized by infection of viscera by the parasite (Chagas' disease); the loss of bowel ganglion cells is a notable feature.

150 E Water is contaminated (B) by human faeces containing cysts of *Entamoeba histolytica*; the cysts release four motile trophozoites in the intestine (D). If these are pathogenic they cause necrosis of intestinal cells (C) and invade the submucosa entering the portal blood stream (E) and resulting in a hepatic abscess (A).

151 If the following events were placed in chronological order which would come
    fourth?
    A. Adult worms migrate to the perivesical veins
    B. Cercaria released from snail
    C. Human epidermis penetrated
    D. Maturation in the portal veins
    E. Miracidia hatch from eggs in fresh water

152 For each of the lesions on the left select the most appropriate parasite from the
    list on the right.
    a. Cyst in the right lobe   A. Echinococcus granulosis
       of the liver   B. Onchocerca volvulus
    b. Elephantiasis   C. Opisthorchis sinensis
    c. Subcutaneous nodules,   D. *Taenia solium*
       blindness   E. Wucheraria bancrofti

151   **D**   Schistosome eggs excreted in faeces or urine hatch out in fresh
water (E) and release miracidia that invade snails; cercaria are
released from the snail (B) and invade human skin (C) losing their
tails. The larva invades vessels, reaches the liver and enters the
portal circulation (D) where it matures and the adults migrate to
the perivesical veins (A). The adults lay eggs, which are excreted
by the host.

152 **a** = **A**   Visceral cysts containing daughter cysts and scolices are the
pathological features of hydatid disease.

b = **E**   In lymphatic filariasis lymphatics are blocked by the adult worms,
giving gross lymphoedema and reactive fibrosis of soft tissues.

c = **B**   Ocular damage due to the presence of the microfilaria in the eye is
the most serious effect ('river blindness').
The adult *Opisthorchis* attaches to the biliary epithelium and may
promote the development of cholangiocarcinoma (C). Man is the
definitive host for *Taenia solium* (the pork tapeworm).

1   The following statements regarding *normal cell structure* are True or False?
    A. Coated vesicles consist of internalised clathrin-coated pits
    B. Microfilaments are composed of actin linked with troponin
    C. Secondary lysosomes are formed by fusion of lysosomes and phagosomes
    D. The low density lipoprotein receptor (LDL) gene is on chromosome 19
    E. The symbiont hypothesis proposes the origin of the nucleus

2   The following statements regarding *irreversible cell injury* are True or False?
    A. Acid hydrolases cause hydrolysis
    B. Free radicals may be removed by vitamin E
    C. Hydroxyl radical is the primary cause of lipid damage
    D. Mitochondrial changes are seen early in cell damage
    E. Reperfusion injury is due to free radical production

3   The following statements regarding *genetic diseases* are True or False?
    A. Autosomal dominant disorders affect twice as many males as females
    B. In autosomal recessive diseases both parents must be heterozygotes
    C. Lyonization accounts for symptomatic female carriers of an X-linked recessive
       disorder
    D. Recessive traits usually result in defective enzymes
    E. Vitamin D resistant rickets is an example of an X-linked dominant condition

4   The following statements regarding *chromosomal disorders* are True or False?
    A. Aneuploidy usually results from non-disjunction
    B. Autosomal trisomy does not produce severe defects
    C. Balanced translocations cause severe abnormalities
    D. Polyploid cells contain an exact multiple of the haploid number
    E. Triploid cells contain three times the diploid number

5   The following statements regarding *types of oedema* are True or False?
    A. Deep venous thrombosis of calf veins is the commonest pathological cause of
       local oedema in the legs
    B. Generalised oedema becomes apparent only when the retained water exceeds
       10l
    C. Generalised oedema due to hypoproteinaemia occurs in the nephrotic
       syndrome
    D. Pulmonary oedema occurs with a slight rise in pulmonary capillary hydrostatic
       pressure
    E. Removal of axillary nodes can cause local oedema of the arm

1 A. **True**   In receptor-mediated endocytosis the ligand binds to the receptor and is internalised to form the coated vesicle, clad in clathrin.

   B. **False** Microfilaments are composed of filamentous actin, which is similar to smooth muscle actin but is not associated with troponin.

   C. **True**   Phagosomes containing ingested material fuse with the primary lysosome to form the secondary lysosome. This process leads to activation of the acid hydrolases in the lysosome.

   D. **True**   This may give insight into the mechanisms involved in familial hypercholesterolaemia, since LDL is rich in cholesterol.

   E. **False** The symbiont hypothesis explains the origin of the mitochondrion on the basis of symbiotic bacteria colonising eukaryotic cells.

2 A. **True**   The release of acid hydrolases from lysosomes results in destruction of intracellular membranes.

   B. **True**   Vitamin E, glutathione and D-penicillamine remove free radicals.

   C. **True**   Hydroxyl radicals react with unsaturated bonds and the resulting product forms a lipid peroxide.

   D. **True**   These are the earliest recognisable ultrastructural changes.

   E. **True**   Following prolonged hypoxic damage restoration of blood supply results in toxic free radical production.

3 A. **False** The numbers are evenly split between male and female. 50% of offspring are affected.

   B. **True**   The parents are unaffected carriers. The risk of further affected children is 1 in 4.

   C. **True**   In X-linked recessive disorders females are carriers as they will have one normal X-chromosome. Non-random inactivation of an X-chromosome (Lyonization) allows the mutant gene to remain active in many cells.

   D. **True**   Recessive traits are usually more severe than dominant traits that result in damage to structural proteins.

   E. **True**   X-linked dominant conditions are very rare, with both male and female affected.

4 A. **True**   The number of chromosomes in an aneuploid cell is not an exact multiple of the haploid number. This may also occur as a result of anaphase lag.

   B. **False** This is usually associated with miscarriage and multiple defects.

   C. **False** There is no loss of DNA, and no clinical abnormality.

   D. **True**

   E. **False** They contain three times the haploid number. This is usually the result of dispermy (fertilization by two sperm)

5 A. **True**   Deep venous thrombosis causes venous obstruction, raising venous hydrostatic pressure.

   B. **False** Fluid retention over 5l will be seen as generalised oedema.

   C. **True**   In the nephrotic syndrome protein, principally albumin, is lost in the urine. Oedema occurs when the level falls below 25 g/l.

   D. **False** Pulmonary capillary hydrostatic pressure (8–10 mmHg) and plasma osmotic pressure (25 mmHg) are widely different. A considerable rise in pulmonary pressure is needed to produce oedema.

   E. **True**   Chronic lymphatic obstruction may occur following radical breast surgery and radiotherapy, and can cause a firm, non-pitting oedema.

6   The following statements regarding *fibrinolysis* are True or False?
    A. Fibrin degradation products (FDP) may be detected in blood and urine
    B. Plasminogen is the most important proteolytic enzyme
    C. Plasminogen and tissue plasminogen activator (t-PA) bind to fibrin
    D. t-PA is synthesized by endothelial cells
    E. Urokinase plasminogen activator (u-PA) binds to specific cell membrane
       receptors

7   The following statements regarding *the action of polymorphs in microbial killing*
    are True or False?
    A. Opsonins promote phagocytosis
    B. Oxygen dependent microbial killing depends on the 'respiratory burst'
    C. Oxygen independent microbial killing is carried out by lysosomal enzymes
    D. Plasma fibronectin is an opsonin
    E. Superoxide dismutase converts superoxide anion to H_2O

8   The following statements regarding *cell derived mediators of the acute
    inflammatory reaction* are True or False?
    A. Glucocorticoids have anti-inflammatory activity because they induce lipocortin
       which inhibits phospholipase A_2
    B. Histamine and serotonin cause vascular dilatation and increase permeability.
    C. PGE_2 causes pain and fever
    D. Phospholipase A_2 is responsible for the release of arachidonic acid from the
       cell membrane
    E. Platelet activating factor (PAF) increases vascular permeability and inhibits
       synthesis of arachidonic acid derivatives

9   The following statements regarding the *acute phase response* are True or False?
    A. Colony stimulating factors (CSFs) are produced by activated T-lymphocytes
    B. Exogenous pyrogens act on leucocytes to produce interleukin-1 (IL-1)
    C. Hepatic protein synthesis is increased in response to infection
    D. PGE_2 is the secondary signal for elevation of body temperature
    E. Tumour necrosis factor (TNF-α) decreases catabolic activity

6 A. **True** FDP's are cleared by the mononuclear phagocyte system which may become saturated allowing FDP's into the blood and urine.
   B. **False** Plasminogen is an inactive pro-enzyme which is converted to plasmin by t-PA and u-PA.
   C. **True** As fibrin is formed in the vessel t-PA and plasminogen bind to it and the activated plasmin degrades the fibrin.
   D. **True** t-PA acts intravascularly; u-PA is extravascular, being produced by various cell types.
   E. **True** Many cells have u-PA surface receptors and this allows extracellular matrix digestion that may be important for tumour invasion, and in embryogenesis.

7 A. **True** Opsonins on the material to be phagocytosed act as ligands for specific cell receptors and promote phagocytosis.
   B. **True** The 'respiratory burst' follows activation of cell membrane NADPH oxidase by phagocytosis, and results in the formation of H_2O_2, superoxide anion and singlet oxygen.
   C. **True** Primary and secondary granules contain enzymes such as lysozyme and myeloperoxidase. This is probably less important than oxygen dependent killing.
   D. **True** Fibronectin, IgG and C3b are all opsonins.
   E. **False** Superoxide dismutase converts superoxide anion to H_2O_2, which is a powerful bactericidal agent that also causes cell injury – it is inactivated by cytoplasmic glutathione peroxidase.

8 A. **True** This results in decreased prostaglandin production. Aspirin acts by inhibiting cyclo-oxygenase activity.
   B. **True** Histamine and serotonin are produced by mast cells, basophils and platelets, and increase permeability via H_1-receptors on post-capillary venules.
   C. **True** PGE_2 is synthesised by macrophages and neutrophils (along with PGD_2 and PGF_2) and also causes vasodilatation.
   D. **True** Phospholipase A_2 releases arachidonic acid from the cell membrane phospholipid and this results in the production of prostaglandins and leukotrienes.
   E. **False** PAF does increase vascular permeability but it stimulates the production of arachidonic acid derivatives.

9 A. **True** Activated T-lymphocytes and macrophages produce CSF's that stimulate the proliferation of myeloid precursors in the bone marrow.
   B. **True** Exogenous pyrogens (e.g. gram-negative bacterial endotoxins) stimulate the production of endogenous pyrogens (IL-1) from leucocytes. IL-1 acts on the thermosensory centres in the anterior hypothalamus.
   C. **False** Hepatic protein synthesis is diminished and the level of serum albumin decreases, while other proteins involved in inflammation rise.
   D. **True** IL-1 acts on the thermoregulatory centre by stimulating formation of PGE_2, which raises the temperature. Aspirin lowers fever by blocking PGE_2 formation.
   E. **False** TNF and IL-1 increase catabolism and hence weight is lost.

10 The following statements regarding *growth factors* are True or False?
    A. Epithelial growth factor (EGF) and transforming growth factor (TGF-α) stimulate epithelial cell regeneration and migration
    B. Fibroblast growth factor (FGF) stimulates endothelial cells
    C. Insulin-like growth factors (IGF-I, IGF-II) are found in the plasma
    D. Platelet derived growth factor (PDGF) stimulates migration of fibroblasts and smooth muscle cells
    E. Transforming growth factor (TGF-β) stimulates epithelial regeneration

11 The following are features of *the specific immune response* – True or False?
    A. Immunological tolerance
    B. Mast cells and basophils
    C. Memory
    D. Secretion of tears
    E. Self/non-self discrimination

12 The following statements are True or False?
    A. An allo-antigen is derived from an identical twin
    B. An auto-antigen is derived from the same species as the host
    C. A hetero-antigen is derived from a species other than the host
    D. An iso-antigen comes from a different inbred strain
    E. A xenograft occurs between individuals of the same species

13 The following statements about the *major histocompatibility complex* are True or False?
    A. Class II antigens are encoded by genes in the HLA-D region
    B. Class II antigens are expressed by resting keratinocytes
    C. Class III region genes encode for proteins involved in the effector arm of the immune response
    D. The chain of class I MHC antigens consists of β_2 microglobulin
    E. The MHC gene complex is found on the short arm of chromosome 7

14 The following associations of *antigens and type 3 hypersensitivity reactions* are True or False?
    A. β-haemolytic streptococci and glomerulonephritis
    B. Gold and membranous nephropathy
    C. Hepatitis B and systemic lupus erythematosis
    D. Streptococcus viridans and bacterial endocarditis
    E. Treponema pallidum and Jarisch-Herxheimer reaction

15 The following statements regarding *transplantation* are True or False?
    A. Chronic graft versus host (GVH) disease resembles autoimmune disease clinically
    B. 'Passenger leucocytes' come from the recipient's bone marrow
    C. The chances of finding an identical sibling are 1:8
    D. Up to 70% of bone marrow recipients develop acute GVH
    E. Vascular endothelium is the major target of the rejection response

10 A. **True** EGF and TGF-α share a common receptor on epithelial cells and may act as paracrine agents.

    B. **True** FGF was initially isolated from brain and pituitary, but stimulates endothelial cells and fibroblasts.

    C. **True** IGFs are similar to a precursor form of insulin and are found in plasma. They are important in embryogenesis (IGF-II) and post-natal development (IGF-I).

    D. **True** PDGF may be important in wound healing. It is found in platelet α-granules.

    E. **False** TGF-β promotes matrix formation by stimulating fibroblast secretion and inhibiting collagenase. It inhibits cell replication.

11 A. **True** Exposure to self components in fetal life leads to a state of specific unresponsiveness.

    B. **False** Mast cells and basophils are part of the non-specific cellular defence mechanism.

    C. **True** Immunological memory is essential for the rapid response to subsequent exposure to antigens.

    D. **False** This is a non-specific defence mechanism.

    E. **True** This is essential to prevent reaction against the body's own tissues. It may become defective resulting in autoimmune disease such as pernicious anaemia.

12 A. **False** An allo-antigen comes from a genetically different individual from within the same species. Identical twins are syngeneic.

    B. **False** An auto-antigen is directed against an antibody from the same individual.

    C. **True**

    D. **True**

    E. **False** A xenograft occurs between inividuals of a different species.

13 A. **True**

    B. **False** Class II antigens are expressed by dendritic cells and B-lymphocytes, and are involved in antigen presentation to T-cells. Some cells, e.g. keratinocytes can express class II antigens if appropriately stimulated, e.g. by interferon.

    C. **True** These genes encode for C4, C2, heat shock protein 70 and TNF.

    D. **True**

    E. **False**   It is on the short arm of chromosome 6.

14 A. **True**

    B. **True**

    C. **False** There is an association with polyarteritis nodosa.

    D. **True**

    E. **True**

15 A. **True** Particularly Sjogren's disease and systemic sclerosis.

    B. **False** 'Passenger leucocytes' are found in the donor tissues. Dendritic cells expressing class I and II MHC are particularly important.

    C. **False** The chance is 1:4 since MHC genes are inherited as extended haplotypes.

    D. **True**

    E. **True** Vascular endothelium is rich in class I and II MHC antigens, which are the main target for rejection.

16 The following are features of the CREST syndrome – True or False?
    A. Calcinosis
    B. Oesophageal involvement
    C. Rheumatoid arthritis
    D. Sclerodactyly
    E. Thrombosis

17 The following are possible mechanisms for the production of autoimmune
    disease – True or False?
    A. Deletion of autoreactive T-cells during ontogeny
    B. Disturbance of the $T_s:T_h$ ratio
    C. Facultative MHC expression
    D. Bypass of T-cell tolerance
    E. Release of sequestered antigen

18 The following statements about the *Human Immunodeficiency Virus (HIV)* are
    True or False?
    A. HIV is closely related to the lentiviruses
    B. Integration of HIV-1 DNA always results in cell death
    C. There are three known strains
    D. The HIV envelope protein gp120 binds to CD4 on B-cells
    E. The viral core contains two protein shells

19 The following statements regarding *AIDS* are True or False?
    A. A rise in CD8+ T-cells is the earliest immunological abnormality
    B. Hypergammaglobulinaemia occurs due to concurrent infections
    C. Kaposi's sarcoma is common in intravenous drug abusers
    D. The best index of disease status is the absolute number of CD8+ T-cells
    E. The main route of transmission is parenteral

20 The following statements regarding *Gaucher's disease* are True or False?
    A. Gaucher cells contain glucocerebroside
    B. Glucocerebroside-β-glucosidase is deficient
    C. It is the commonest lysosomal storage disorder
    D. Osteonecrosis may occur
    E. Type II has the best prognosis

16 A. **True**
     B. **True**
     C. **False**   Raynaud's phenomenon.
     D. **True**
     E. **False**   Telangiectasia.
                  The CREST syndrome is one type of systemic sclerosis in which there is cutaneous and visceral involvement. In progressive systemic sclerosis there is extensive visceral involvement.

17 A. **False**   During ontogeny most autoreactive lymphocytes (mostly T-cells) are deleted. A possible mechanism for autoimmune disease is a defect in this deletion process allowing autoreactive cells to exist in adult life.
     B. **True**
     C. **True**   In most organ-specific autoimmune diseases there is aberrant expression of class II HLA molecules on the target cells.
     D. **True**
     E. **True**

18 A. **True**   HIV is structurally similar to the lentiviruses, e.g. feline and simian immunodeficiency viruses which cause similar clinical disease in cats and monkeys.
     B. **False**   Productive infection leads to cell death, but some cells with integrated HIV and DNA do not suffer cytopathic effects until the T-cell is activated, perhaps by concurrent viral infection.
     C. **False**   There are two strains: HIV-1 (North America, Europe, Central Africa) and HIV-2 (West Africa).
     D. **False**   The CD4 antigen is on T-cells and is the receptor for the gp120 viral envelope protein, allowing HIV to infect T-cells.
     E. **True**   The core consists of an outer protein shell (p18) and an inner protein shell (p24). The RNA genome and reverse transcriptase are within the inner shell.

19 A. **True**   This occurs at the time of seroconversion.
     B. **True**   Polyclonal B-cell activation may be a result of infection by other viruses, e.g. cytomegalovirus, Epstein-Barr virus.
     C. **False**   Kaposi's sarcoma occurs mainly in homosexual and bisexual males.
     D. **False**   The absolute numbers of CD4+ T-cells is the best index.
     E. **False**   Venereal transmission is the major route worldwide.

20 A. **True**   Gaucher cells are 20–100 μm diameter cells with fibrillary cytoplasm containing strands of glucocerebroside.
     B. **True**
     C. **True**
     D. **True**   Hepatosplenomegaly, anaemia, flaring of the metaphyses of long bones and osteonecrosis are all features of the chronic (Type I) disease.
     E. **False**   This has the worst prognosis as there is no residual enzyme activity. Death occurs in infancy.

21   The following statements regarding *phenylketonuria* are True or False?
     A. Conversion of phenylalanine to tyrosine is inhibited
     B. The enzyme defect is phenylalanine 4-mono-oxygenase
     C. The incidence in the United Kingdom is 190 per million live births
     D. There is a prenatal test available
     E. Treatment is by diet

22   The following statements regarding *cystic fibrosis* are True or False?
     A. Affects 1:2000 live births
     B. Heterozygous carrier prevalence is 1:25
     C. Sweat chloride levels > 60 mmol/l are diagnostic
     D. The gene is on the long arm of chromosome 9
     E. The most common CF gene mutation is deletion of the codon for phenylalanine

23   The following statements regarding the *bacterial cell wall* are True or False?
     A. Cholesterol is part of the cytoplasmic membrane
     B. Flagella originate in the cytoplasmic membrane
     C. Gram-positive bacteria have a thick peptidoglycan layer
     D. Mesosomes have a similar function to mitochondria
     E. The porin is responsible for the transport of hydrophobic molecules

24   The following statements regarding *bacterial pathogenicity* are True or False?
     A. Aggressins are exotoxins
     B. Endotoxins are produced by gram-positive bacteria
     C. Exotoxins are heat stable at 100° C
     D. Fimbriate strains adhere to mucosal epithelial cells
     E. Invasiveness often depends on ability to resist phagocytosis

25   The following are functions of the *virion* – True or False?
     A. Acts as a structural package for the genome
     B. Contains RNA and DNA
     C. May carry transcriptase enzymes
     D. Protects the viral genome from UV-irradiation
     E. Surface proteins bind to target cell receptors

26   The following are *effects of starvation* – True or False?
     A. Adipose tissue releases free fatty acids
     B. Hypoglycaemia
     C. Ketone bodies utilised as a source of energy
     D. Muscle glycogen mobilized
     E. Muscle protein broken down

21 A. **True**
    B. **True**
    C. **True**   Elsewhere it is nearer 100 per million.
    D. **False**   The Guthrie test is performed on blood removed postnatally. Linkage analysyis of DNA restriction fragment length polymorphism may be useful in families already known to carry the defect.
    E. **True**   Dietary exclusion of phenylalanine is essential. It may be possible to return to a normal diet after the age of 10.

22 A. **True**
    B. **True**
    C. **True**   Elevated sodium and chloride in the sweat are easily detected. Secretion is normal but the chloride is not reabsorbed by the cells of the sweat duct.
    D. **False**   It is on the long arm of chromosome 7 (7q31).
    E. **True**

23 A. **False**   The cytoplasmic membrane consists of structural and enzymic proteins in a phospholipid bilayer.
    B. **True**   These are found on bacilli but not cocci.
    C. **True**   In gram-positive bacteria there is a thick peptidoglycan layer containing teichoic acid. It is the structure of this layer that is responsible for the staining characteristics.
    D. **True**   Mesosomes are involved in DNA segregation during cell division. They also contain respiratory enzymes.
    E. **False**   Hydrophilic molecules are transported across the porins.

24 A. **True**   Aggressins are exotoxins that increase bacterial ability to penetrate and multiply. *Staphylococcus aureus* coagulase is an example.
    B. **False**   Endotoxins are produced by gram-negative bacteria.
    C. **False**   Exotoxins are usually inactivated by heating to 70–100° C. Endotoxins are heat stable.
    D. **True**   The presence of fimbria is helpful in increasing bacterial adhesion to epithelial cells. P-fimbria are mannose resistant fimbria on *Escheria coli* that cause urinary tract infections.
    E. **True**   Invasiveness often depends on the ability to avoid phagocytosis, e.g. *Staphylococcus aureus* produces protein A.

25 A. **True**
    B. **False**   It contains either RNA or DNA.
    C. **True**   Negative-sense single-stranded RNA genomes require transcriptase to initiate host manufacture of complementary RNA copies.
    D. **True**   This is essential during host to host transfer.
    E. **True**   Influenza virus haemagglutinin protein binds to receptors on respiratory epithelium.

26 A. **True**   Increased fat catabolism releases free fatty acids, which are used as an energy source.
    B. **True**   Glucose is used up as an energy substrate.
    C. **True**   Fatty acid metabolism produces ketone bodies which accumulate since the citric acid cycle is impaired. These ketone bodies are used as an energy source, especially by the brain.
    D. **False**   Muscle glycogen is not used since muscle lacks glucose-6-phosphatase. Hepatic glycogen is broken down to glucose.
    E. **True**   Muscle protein is broken down to release amino acids that are incorporated in hepatic gluconeogenesis.

27 The following statements regarding *cell cycle control* are True or False?
   A. Mitosis promoting factor (MPF) is responsible for the transition from G2 to M phase
   B. p34 is phosphorylated prior to M phase
   C. p34 kinase is a component of MPF
   D. Phosphorylated cyclin B is essential for entry to mitosis
   E. Protein product of c-*srs* is partially responsible for the changes in cell shape

28 The following are features of the *transformed phenotype* – True or False?
   A. Cells grow in parallel arrays *in vitro*
   B. Fails to show topo-inhibition (contact inhibition)
   C. Forms colonies in suspension culture
   D. Growth is dependent on additional growth factors
   E. Proliferation in confluent culture

29 The following factors are *possible mechanisms for invasion by tumour cells* – True or False?
   A. Tumour cells produce defective basement membrane
   B. Tumour cells bind more weakly to tenascin than to fibronectin
   C. Tumour cells secrete tissue inhibitors of metalloproteases (TIMP)
   D. Tumour cells stimulate the secretion of stromelysin 3
   E. Tumour cells release type IV collagenase

30 The following statements regarding *tissue damage by radiation* are True or False?
   A. Cataract occurs with a dose greater than 6Gy
   B. Hair loss is permanent with a dose of 6Gy
   C. Type II pneumocyte proliferation is responsible for acute radiation pneumonitis
   D. Testicular germ cells are less sensitive than Sertoli cells
   E. The severity of diarrhoea is a good predictor of chronic intestinal radiation damage

27 A. **True**   MPF is a heterodimer consisting of p34 kinase and cyclin B.
    B. **False** p34 is dephosphorylated just before mitosis.
    C. **True**
    C. **True**   Cyclin B is phosphorylated at the same time as p34 is dephosphorylated and the complex of the two initiates mitosis.
    D. **True**   c-*src*, histone, lamin and caldesmon are all substrates of p34 kinase.

28 A. **True**
    B. **True**
    C. **False** Tumour cells do not require additional growth factors as non-neoplastic cells do to continue growth in culture.
    D. **False** Tumour cells characteristically grow in a haphazard way overlapping one another in culture.
    E. **True**

29 A. **True**
    B. **False** Tumour cells alter the extracellular matrix; tenascin is found in high concentration in the stroma of some tumours (breast particularly), and it binds tumour cells less effectively than fibronectin.
    C. **False** Normal tissues contain TIMP's; tumour cells may secrete inhibitors of TIMP's.
    D. **True**   Stromal cells are stimulated by PDGF and TGF secreted by tumour cells to secrete stromelysin 3.
    E. **True**   Basement membrane consists largely of type IV collagen.

30 A. **True**
    B. **False** A dose greater than 40Gy is required.
    C. **True**
    D. **False** The germ cells are more sensitive than the Sertoli cells. In females the follicular granulosa cells are more sensitive than the germ cells.
    E. **True**